D0091118

THE DIABETES TRAVEL GUIDE

2ND EDITION

How to travel with diabetes—anywhere in the world

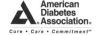

American Diabetes Association.
Cure • Care • Commitment™

DAVIDA F. KRUGER, MSN, APRN-BC, BC-ADM

Director, Book Publishing, John Fedor; *Managing Editor, Book Publishing,* Abe Ogden; *Acquisitions Editor, Consumer Books,* Robert Anthony; *Production Manager,* Melissa Sprott; *Composition,* ADA; *Cover Design,* Pixiedesign; *Printer,* Transcontinental Printing.

Printed in Canada
1 3 5 7 9 10 8 6 4 2

The suggestions and information contained in this publication are generally consistent with the Clinical Practice Recommendations and other policies of the American Diabetes Association, but they do not represent the policy or position of the Association or any of its boards or committees. Reasonable steps have been taken to ensure the accuracy of the information presented. However, the American Diabetes Association cannot ensure the safety or efficacy of any product or service described in this publication. Individuals are advised to consult a physician or other appropriate health care professional before undertaking any diet or exercise program or taking any medication referred to in this publication. Professionals must use and apply their own professional judgment, experience, and training and should not rely solely on the information contained in this publication before prescribing any diet, exercise, or medication. The American Diabetes Association—its officers, directors, employees, volunteers, and members—assumes no responsibility or liability for personal or other injury, loss, or damage that may result from the suggestions or information in this publication.

⊛ The paper in this publication meets the requirements of the ANSI Standard Z39.48-1992 (permanence of paper).

ADA titles may be purchased for business or promotional use or for special sales. To purchase more than 50 copies of this book at a discount, or for custom editions of this book with your logo, contact Lee Romano Sequeira, Special Sales & Promotions, at the address below, or at LRomano@diabetes.org or 703-299-2046. For all other inquiries, please call 1-800-DIABETES.

American Diabetes Association
1701 North Beauregard Street
Alexandria, Virginia 22311

Library of Congress Cataloging-in-Publication Data

Kruger, Davida F., 1954-
  The diabetes travel guide / Davida Kruger. -- 2nd ed.
     p. cm.
  Includes bibliographical references and index.
  ISBN-13: 978-1-58040-236-1 (alk. paper)
  1. Diabetes--Popular works. 2. Travel--Health aspects--Popular works. I. Title.

  RC660.4.K784 2006
  616.4'62--dc22

                              2006018455

To Brianne, Andrea, and Leah, who never cease to bring joy to my life,

And

Fred W. Whitehouse, MD, who has taught me to seek what the color blue implies.

CONTENTS

PREFACE

My mother was diagnosed with diabetes at the age of 30. The 17 years she lived with diabetes were challenging. It was the era before self-monitoring of blood glucose and before we understood the importance of good diabetes control.

In 1982, the year my mother died, I completed my graduate work. I was hired by Fred W. Whitehouse, MD, as a Nurse Practitioner and began my career in diabetes. Through his never-ending support and guidance, I have remained in that position at Henry Ford Health System.

Over the past 25 years, our knowledge of diabetes and of the best care and treatment has changed. However, the disease continues to challenge all who are touched by it. It is my hope that this book will help in some way.

I thank my patients and their families for sharing their knowledge and experiences that added a personal touch and depth to this book. I thank Gayle Lorenzi for her review of the manuscript. And I thank my family for allowing me the solitude needed to complete this book and for their ongoing support.

Chapter One

PREPARING FOR YOUR TRIP

Whether you're going across the state or around the world, the best approach to travel is to be prepared. And if you have diabetes, that's the only way to travel. Plan for as much of the trip as you can. Be curious and ask lots of questions. Questions are the beginning of your "quest" and of being adventurous. Ask questions of health care providers, friends with diabetes who travel, travel agents, and, if you can, people who have been to the location you're going to visit. Try to learn all about the area. Be ready for the unexpected, including cancelled flights, lost luggage, and illness. Do not assume that you will be able to buy your diabetes supplies when you get there. Take what you need and then pack extra. Picture yourself as a prepared and capable traveler, and get ready to have fun!

DO YOUR RESEARCH

Local libraries and bookstores have many travel books to help you choose and learn more about your destination—climate, terrain, wildlife, culture, foods, and other points of interest. Check out the internet and find out more about the places you want to visit. Many destinations also have tourism councils that will be happy to provide you with as much information as they can. And remember, never be afraid to ask friends, relatives, coworkers, acquaintances, online forum members, or anyone else who may have already blazed this path ahead of you. First-person information can often be the most useful. You may have been learning about the place you want to visit for many years, but once you decide to go, start preparing several months in advance.

Researching travel online

These days, it's hard to imagine planning a vacation or trip without the internet. Almost any travel information a person could need is available online. If you do not own a computer, the local library will probably have computers you can use.

On the Web

There are thousands of websites for travelers, so look around. Throughout this book we try to mention as many helpful websites as we can. Here are a couple of good places to start.

www.diabetes.org

This is the website for the American Diabetes Association and it is easily the most comprehensive and reliable resource for diabetes information on the web. Here you can find information on nutrition, medication, breaking news, policy, insurance, and much more. There's even a community forum for people with diabetes from around the world to gather to discuss diabetes online.

www.lonelyplanet.com

This is the website of the comprehensive Lonely Planet series of travel books. If there is a place humans can visit, Lonely Planet probably publishes a travel book covering it.

Many states and countries have their own web pages with information about the area and special events. An area's Convention and Visitor's Bureau (CVB) can also provide much information.

The internet can also help you with find a hotel. Once you have decided where to stay, take a virtual tour of the hotel on the internet. This may help you get a better feel for the facilities and let you see what types of amenities, dining options, and nearby attractions are available. Once you have decided on a hotel, you can request an email address to ask pre-trip questions.

SEE YOUR PROVIDER EARLY

At least 4–6 weeks before your trip, see your health care provider. You need to schedule this visit far enough in advance so your provider can help you plan. This is a good time to

- have a physical exam;
- look at how well your diabetes program is working;

- make a plan for sick days if you don't already have one;
- talk about foot care;
- discuss any letters and documents you will need on your travels (see below).

Discuss your travel plans in detail and ask questions that may save you a lot of frustration (or worse) later. Also get extra prescriptions for your diabetes medications and supplies that you can carry with you.

A letter from your health care provider

Ask your health care provider to write a letter for you stating that you have diabetes and you must have your diabetes supplies with you at all times (see *Example of a Diabetes Letter*). This letter comes in very handy, for example, if you have to explain to customs officials why you are carrying syringes. Or if you are observing a debate from the seats overlooking the Senate floor in Washington, D.C., take out your meter to check your blood glucose, and are abruptly removed from the area by guards who do not know what your meter is.

Be sure you request this letter far enough in advance so that your health care provider can prepare it for you. Do not expect to leave your health care providers office with the letter in hand on the day of your visit. The letter from your provider should state

- that you have diabetes;
- your insulin and other injectable or oral medication program;
- if possible, the adjustments to make for sick days;
- if possible, the phone number of health care facilities or providers in the area you will be traveling through.

! Carry a copy of your diabetes letters with you at all times.

You should also carry a prescription or letter with information about the insulin, other injectable medications and syringes, or oral diabetes medications you use (see *Example of a Prescription Letter*). The second letter should state (and you should know) the types of insulin, the concentration (U-100), the dose(s), and the size of your insulin syringe (see Table 3-1). For diabetes pills, the letter should state the type(s) of pills (see Table 4-1 on page 99), how often to take them, how much to take, and whether they can cause you to have low blood glucose.

You should make several photocopies of both of these letters and carry a copy of each with you at all times.

FOR HELP WHEN YOU GET THERE

Before traveling, you can call ahead to the convention and visitors' bureau of the state or country for help in locating health care facilities in the area where you will be traveling. Your health care providers also may be able to provide you with the name and

> ## On the Web
> ### www.istm.org
> Website for the International Society of Travel Medicine, this site provides in-depth health and safety profiles of countries around the world. The Society also publishes a list of health care providers in foreign cities, though it does not rate or endorse any provider.

Example of a Diabetes Letter

Date:

To Whom It May Concern:

RE: (*Your Name*)

(*Your Name*) has diabetes mellitus. As part of his diabetes regimen, it is necessary for him to take insulin (and/or names of other injectable medications) and monitor his blood glucose daily. When traveling, he must carry insulin, insulin syringes, a blood glucose meter, and lancets.

If you have any questions regarding his diabetes care or the supplies he carries with him, please feel free to contact me.

Sincerely yours,

(*Provider's signature*)

Health care provider name:

_____

Address:

_____

Telephone numbers:

_____

phone number of a hospital or clinic and provider in the area.

In the United States, the American Diabetes Association (ADA) can direct you to health care professionals who participate in recognized diabetes education programs and provider recognition programs. These health care providers all follow ADA standards of care. You can call 1-800-DIABETES (1-800-342-2383) or visit *www.diabetes.org* for more information and referrals to health care professionals in the areas you will be visiting.

TAKE YOUR PRESCRIPTIONS WITH YOU

In addition to taking your diabetes supplies with you (and packing extra), be sure to take a copy of the prescription for each of your medications and needed supplies in case you need more. Ask your provider to write the prescriptions for the generic brand, especially when you plan to travel out of the country. This will make it easier for you to find the medications, since most medications have different trade names throughout the world.

Example of a Prescription Letter

Date:

To Whom It May Concern:

RE: (*Your Name*)

(*Your Name*) has diabetes mellitus. Her present insulin program requires her to take two injections of insulin daily. Her breakfast dose of insulin is 42 units of NPH human insulin and 18 units of lispro (generic of both). Before dinner, she takes 46 units of NPH human insulin and 22 units of rapid-acting analog. In addition, she takes Symlin (pramlintide), 20 units injected before meals. The insulin is U-100. She uses a 1-cc, 29-gauge, 1/2" insulin syringe. If you have any questions regarding her diabetes care, please feel free to contact me.

Sincerely,

(*Provider's signature*)

Health care provider name:

_____

Address:

_____

Telephone numbers:

_____

If you're traveling within the United States, call ahead to see whether pharmacies in the state you are traveling to will accept prescriptions from a different state. If you are taking a newly approved medication, you may want to ask if the local pharmacy carries it; sometimes pharmacies do not stock new medications and have to order them. If this is the case, you may need to wait for several days. Finding a pharmacy that carries your prescribed medications is important. This is usually not a problem, but checking it out ahead of time may save you time and frustration when you get there.

If you get your prescription from a chain pharmacy, such as CVS or Walgreen's, the prescriptions and your insurance information are kept in a computer database that can be accessed at any of their stores nationwide. Usually, the hotel or facility in which you're staying will have a list of pharmacies in the area. You can call ahead to get this list or ask for it when you arrive.

You need a prescription to purchase oral diabetes medications. However, with the exception of rapid-acting insulins, many

Example of a Letter for Byetta

Date:

To Whom It May Concern:

RE: (*Your Name*)

(*Your Name*) has diabetes mellitus. In addition to the oral medication she takes for her diabetes, she also uses an injectable pen to take Byetta (exenetide), 10 units twice daily.

It is necessary for her to carry both the injectable pen device and pen needles. If you have any questions regarding her diabetes care, please feel free to contact me.

Sincerely,

(*Provider's signature*)

Health care provider name:

_____

Address:

_____

Telephone numbers:

_____

states do not require that you have a prescription to purchase insulin or blood glucose supplies. Keep in mind that when you purchase insulin or blood glucose supplies without a prescription, your insurance does not cover the cost, and you will have to pay full price for the items rather than just your insurance copay.

HEALTH INSURANCE KNOW-HOW

Whether you are traveling out of the state or out of the country, know how your health insurance works. Many health insurance companies will cover the cost of health care throughout the United States.

Warning! Prescriptions Outside of the United States

When you travel to foreign countries, you probably will not be able to get your prescription filled. Make sure you have enough insulin or medication before you leave the country. If something does happen and you need medication, insulin, or supplies, have a prescription with the generic name of your medication on it; this will make it much easier for another physician to help you get the correct medication.

Some companies will only pay for emergency health care in the United States, but you must call a toll-free phone number at the time of care or shortly after for approval. If you are traveling out of the country, it is important to know whether your health insurance will cover emergency health care. Medicare will not cover health care outside of the United States. If you need coverage, you may contact a travel agent to learn about supplemental health care insurance for the time you are on your trip. Some companies also provide insurance for lost baggage and other things that might disrupt your trip.

On the Web

www.international-SOS.com

This is a great website for international travelers looking for insurance information for overseas travel, including paying for your trip home if you become ill.

VACCINES TO KEEP YOU HEALTHY

If you are traveling out of the country, find out if you need vaccines or booster shots. Some vaccines have to be given in a series over several weeks or months, so begin early enough to complete the series. Be sure your tetanus booster is up to date. Then if you get an injury while traveling, it will be one less thing about which you need to be concerned.

Always take a record of your booster shots and vaccines with you when you travel— another of your important papers! Be aware that not all health care providers have these vaccines in their offices. For instance, your diabetes care or primary health care provider may not be able to provide these vaccines for you. So in addition to finding out what vaccines you will

What Vaccines Do You Need?

The Centers for Disease Control and Prevention (CDC) can provide you with a list of the vaccines that travelers need. Call the CDC hotline at 1-877-FYI-TRIP or use their website at *www.cdc.gov* to determine what shots you may need for the locations you want to visit. Or you can call a local hospital and ask for their Department of Health Travel or Infectious Diseases. People in these departments can tell you what vaccines you need.

need, be sure to find out where you can get them.

PASSPORTS AND VISAS

A passport is an official document stating that you are a citizen of a certain country. It is necessary to have one if you plan to travel outside the United States. In addition to a passport, some countries also require that you get a visa before visiting. Obtaining a passport and a visa takes time, so once you know you will be traveling outside the country, start the paperwork. It's worth the effort to get the application into the mail at least 6–8 weeks ahead of time, because it is much easier to obtain these documents through the mail.

How to get a passport

To obtain or renew your passport in the United States, you will need to fill out an application. These can be found at the following locations in your area:

- Post office
- Court house

- Public library
- Clerk of the court office
- Online at *www.travel.state.gov*

Along with the application, you will need to submit proof of your U.S. citizenship—usually a birth certificate—valid identification, and two identical 2 1/2" by 2 1/2" passport photos of yourself. The application will tell you where to submit the application. As of this printing, the total cost of a passport for new applicants is $97 for those 16 years of age and older and $82 for those under 16. The cost for renewing a passport is $67, and you must send in your old one.

You may use the National Passport Information Center at 1-877-487-2778 to assist you in applying for a passport. A live operator is available Monday through Friday, 7:00 AM–12:00 midnight Eastern Standard Time, except holidays, and the information is available in both English and Spanish. The center can answer questions such as where to apply, how to apply, how to complete the application, the status of your application, and other

On the Web

www.travel.state.gov

This is the travel section of the U.S. State Department website and it's an excellent resource for international travelers. In addition to passport applications and information, you can find information on visas, current travel warnings, and legal issues that may pertain to your travels abroad.

questions you might have. They can also locate the passport office closest to you and schedule an appointment. When operators are not available, there is a 24-hour, 7-day-per-week interactive phone system.

If you need your passport in less than 25 calendar days, call the National Passport Information Center at the number listed above. They will assist you in obtaining your passport. In addition to the other requirements, you will need to send a photocopy of your paid round-trip airplane or boat tickets to show the reason you need the expedited services. Your passport can be sent to you as quickly as 3 business days after the application arrives in the Passport Services office. There is a $60.00 additional fee for express service.

It is also important to note that travel to some countries that once did not require passports from the United States—such as Canada, Mexico, and the Caribbean—may now require a passport. You may also need one for boarding a cruise liner depending on the various ports you will visit. If you're leaving the United States, it is best to have a passport so that your vacation is not ruined.

What's a visa?

A visa is a stamp of official approval from a foreign government that is put in your passport. A visa shows that you are allowed

International Travel Hotline

If you'll be traveling internationally, you might consider calling the Office of Overseas Citizens Services traveler's hotline at 1-202-647-5225. This division of the State Department allows you to register your travel and determine any important information about the country to which you are traveling.

to enter the foreign country, your papers are in order, and the purpose of your trip has been approved. Check with your travel agent, the airlines, or the embassy of the country you will be visiting to find out whether you need a visa. You may also call the National Passport Information Center at 1-877-487-277 or visit *www.travel.state.gov*. Each of these offices can help you determine entry requirements for the country you wish to visit. European countries do not require visas.

MEDICAL IDENTIFICATION

If for some reason you are unable to take care of yourself or speak for yourself, it is very important for those around you to quickly determine that you have diabetes and that you need immediate care. Wearing a medical alert bracelet or necklace can be very helpful in these types of situations. Carrying an identification card in your wallet may also be helpful. However, wearing medical ID is preferable, since there can be times when you are separated from your wallet.

There are many manufacturers producing various types of medical ID, ranging from platinum necklaces to thick leather cuffs.

Look around; there's bound to be something out there you like. Below are a few places to start.

Medical Identification

IdentiFind
1-828-648-6768
www.identifind.com

Medic Alert
1-888-633-4298
www.medicalert.org

Lifetag Medical ID Products
1-888-543-3824
www.lifetag.com

SOS America
1-800-999-1264
www.sosamerica.com

LifeWear
1-415-867-9327
www.mylifewear.com

Goldware Medical Jewelry
1-800-669-7311
www.goldware-id.com

Chapter Two

PACKING FOR YOUR TRIP

Packing the correct items (the ones you'll need) for your trip depends on where you will be going and what you will be doing. The climate and your activities will determine what type of clothes to bring. In addition to clothing, of course, you will pack your diabetes supplies, snacks, and items for an emergency.

If you think through your trip and plan what you may need ahead of time, it always pays off in the long run. You can write down as much of your schedule as you know for each day of your trip and then match your clothing to the schedule. At the same time, you should write down

> ## On the Web
>
> ### *www.travelhealth.com*
>
> This website can make planning and packing for your trip much easier. It discusses water purity, travel illness, treatments, traveling with medications, and pre-travel checklists.

any other items that come to mind so you won't forget to bring them. A checklist is a great help. You may also want to make a checklist of all your medications, devices, and supplies, even if it seems silly. In the frenzy of packing, you won't want to forget needles for your insulin pen or blood glucose strips for your meter. You can keep the lists that work well and use them for future trips.

WHICH SUITCASE?

It is wise to pick the right suitcase for your trip ahead of time. If you will be taking dress clothes, a duffel bag may not be the best choice. Instead, you may prefer to use a garment bag that allows you to hang up suits or dresses. Conversely, if you are traveling to an area where you will be wearing shorts, T-shirts, and a bathing suit, a duffel bag might be just perfect. A suitcase with wheels is also a good idea. Although wheels make a suitcase heavier, rolling a suitcase is easier than trying to carry it. A small tote or backpack is also helpful along the trip and when you arrive at your destination. A tote or backpack provides an easy way to carry diabetes supplies, snacks, travel papers, maps, a camera, and other supplies each day.

Be sure to label each piece of luggage with your name and a phone number. You may want to use a business address on your luggage tag rather than your home address. If someone finds your luggage, you may not want that person to show up at your home unannounced. If you have some type of unusual or colorful tag on your luggage, it'll be easier to spot on the baggage carousel and less likely that someone will take your bag by mistake.

PACKING TWICE

It is important to pack twice as much diabetes medication and supplies as you think you will need. The extra supplies will come in handy if you become ill, some get lost, or other problems arise.

Never pack your diabetes supplies in the luggage that you are going to check. Keep all diabetes supplies and medications with you at all times. If your luggage does not arrive with you, you may need to buy a toothbrush and some new clothes, but you will have your diabetes supplies and medications. If you are traveling with a companion, pack half of your supplies in that person's carry-on bags just in case something happens to yours. It's wise to make a list of the things that belong in your Diabetes Survival Kit (see page 69) to be sure you remember to bring everything you need.

> ! Always pack twice as much medication
> . and supplies as you think you'll need.
>
> ! Keep your diabetes medications and sup-
> . plies with you at all times.

PACKING FOOD

Be sure to pack supplies to treat low blood glucose and plenty of healthy snack foods. These are as important as your medications. Travel may be delayed. Airlines rarely serve meals. Many no longer even provide pretzels with your beverage. Food on the road is often unhealthy. Carrying several nutritious snacks, such as health bars, fruit, or packets of crackers and cheese, can be a great help along the way (see the box *Travel Snacks to Carry*).

Put snacks in zip-top plastic bags to keep them fresh. Many snacks can be purchased in single servings, but this may be more expensive. Read the labels to see how much carbohydrate is in a serving of the food. To treat low blood glucose, you need 15 g of carbohydrate. In addition to the snacks listed in the *Travel Snacks to Carry* box, consider bringing the following:

- One full meal, such as a sandwich, fruit, and dessert
- Single-serving snacks, cereal, or fruit
- Crackers
- Bread
- Chips
- Plastic bowl, plastic utensils

Travel Snacks to Carry	
Snacks	Serving Size (15 g carb)
Animal crackers	7
Ginger snaps	3
Gold fish, pretzels	1/2 cup
Graham crackers	3
Gummy bears	6
Vanilla wafers	5
Oyster crackers	26
Popcorn cakes	2
Pretzel sticks	35
Pretzel rods	2 1/2
Saltines	6
Granola bars	1/2
Single-serving boxes of cereal	1–2
Cheese and cracker packs	1 1/2
Gold fish, cheese (1-oz pack)	1
Raisins	2 Tbsp

If you have dinner at a restaurant, ask for a take-out glass of milk. You can keep it cool on ice or in a hotel mini-bar refrigerator until bedtime. Use it for a bowl of cereal or as part of a bedtime snack.

Unless you are flying first class, meals are rarely served on flights. Be sure to pack a meal or buy one in the airport before you take off. Flights can be delayed even after you board the airplane. If you have planned ahead and brought your own food, you will not have any problems with low blood glucose from a missed meal.

PACKING YOUR TRUSTY MONITOR

Pack extra blood glucose monitoring supplies. If you run out or lose them, you'll need to know the name of your blood glucose monitor, the blood glucose test strips to use with it, and the type of battery. Write this information down and put it with your important travel papers. Also write down the toll-free phone number of the manufacturer of your monitor. Most companies will ship you a new meter wherever you are if yours malfunctions while it is still under warranty. Whenever possible, take a second blood glucose meter with you to use as a backup.

Your insurance company will not purchase a second meter for you, however, so ask your health care providers or pharmacist about special rebate programs. Many companies have rebate programs that will allow you to purchase a second meter at a relatively low cost.

As an emergency backup, if you are going to a wilderness area or someplace you could not get a new battery or replacement for your meter, you might want to carry some visual test strips. These work by putting a drop of blood on the strip and comparing the results to a color chart. This is not nearly as accurate as using a blood glucose meter, but it is better than not having a way to check your blood glucose at all. A more accurate (and more expensive) method worth considering would be to take a Sidekick Testing System (Home Diagnostics, Inc.). The meter is actually built into the top of the vial of 50 strips. When the strips are gone, the entire vial is disposed of.

WHAT ELSE DO YOU PUT IN YOUR CARRY-ON BAG?

A carry-on bag that you keep with you at all times makes sense whether you are flying, driving, or traveling by boat or train.

Once again, you should always keep all of your diabetes medications, supplies, and snacks with you. If the bags you check do not make it to your destination, you will still be able to take care of your diabetes. If you have room in the carry-on bag, you may wish to pack clothing for one day, along with books or magazines to read while you travel.

Occasionally, certain airline security situations place restrictions on various carry-on items; sometimes carry-on bags are prohibited completely. If traveling by air, make sure you have your letters from your doctor and your prescriptions with you at all times. Explain to airport security that

On the Web

www.tsa.gov

This is the website for the U.S. Travel Security Administration and it is packed with information on travel security, including safety measures for traveling (land, sea, and air), the current list of prohibited items for airline travel, the steps to take for help with lost or missing luggage, and much more. This information can also be accessed through their toll-free general contact hotline at 1-866-289-9673.

you have diabetes and that you absolutely need to take a carry-on bag with you onto the plane. Even when security is tight, there are exceptions for those with diabetes and, with the proper documents, getting your supplies and medicine with you onto the plane should not be difficult.

Many of the same security measures that restrict carry-on luggage also restrict specific items, such as nail clippers, scissors, and fluids. If possible, pack a bottle of water, lip balm, and hand cream. These can help you feel more comfortable, but they're non-essential and not worth the trouble during times of heightened security. If you can't carry on fluids, bring an empty water bottle that can be filled on the plane. On long trips, you may feel better taking out your contact lenses and wearing your glasses. Travel papers, passports, and maps also belong in your carry-on bag.

It's wise to keep a light sweater or jacket with you when you travel in case it gets cool. Many airlines no longer provide pillows. If a pillow is important to your comfort, you may wish to purchase a travel pillow to take with you.

Carry-On Rule of Thumb

When trying to determine what should go in your carry-on bag and what should go in checked luggage, keep the following in mind: As long as it is not prohibited by airport security, any item you find useful while traveling or that you would be lost without should be in your carry-on bag.

For the sun

If you will be spending time in the sun, whether on a beach, hiking, or skiing, pack sunscreen. Test the sunscreen before you travel to be sure it will not cause a skin rash or irritation. Eye protection from the sun's rays is also important. Be sure to pack sunglasses or ski goggles.

Some medications can cause problems for you if you are in the sun, and it is difficult to predict when sensitivity to the sun will occur (see the box *Medications that May Cause Sun Sensitivity*). You should use a sunscreen that blocks UV rays if you are taking any medications that can cause you to be sensitive to light (photosensitivity). Your health care provider or pharmacist can advise you about which of your

Medications that May Cause Sun Sensitivity

- Antihistamines
- Coal tar products (such as tegrin and denorex)
- Oral contraceptives and estrogen
- Anti-inflammatory drugs (such as ibuprofen and naproxen)
- Phenothiazines (tranquilizers such as thorazine)
- Sulfa antibiotics (such as bactrim and septra)
- Thiazide diuretics (such as dyazide)
- Tetracycline antibiotics (such as minocycline)
- Tricyclic antidepressants (elavil is used for painful neuropathy)

This list is not final. Review your medications with your pharmacist or health care provider to determine whether any medications you are taking could cause you to be sensitive to the sun.

medications can cause a reaction to the sun and tell you when you should try to stay out of the sun.

Your own first aid kit

Put together a first aid kit for traveling. Be prepared for small emergencies or illnesses with the medications that you might need. If you are leaving the country, take items that will help you if you get one of the common traveler's illnesses. The items in the box *First Aid Kit* are good to have with you.

+ First Aid Kit +

- Bandage tape 1"
- Band-aids
- Gauze pads (4"×4")
- ABD pads (2 large gauze pads)
- Roll of gauze (Kling)
- Ace bandages 2" and 3"
- Butterfly tapes (work like stitches to hold a cut together)
- Tongue depressors (good splints)
- Analgesics (aspirin or acetaminophen)
- Thermometer
- Sunscreen
- Nasal decongestant
- Nose spray
- Tweezers

- Fingernail clipper
- Toenail clipper
- Foil-wrapped sterile wipes
- Antibiotic cream
- Antiseptic (alcohol or betadine)
- Cold pack
- Scissors
- Insect repellent
- Calamine lotion (for insect bites, poison ivy, and sunburn)
- Motion sickness pills
- Glucagon kit (if you take insulin or a diabetes pill that can cause hypoglycemia)
- Pepto Bismol
- Immodium (for diarrhea)
- Sugar-free cough syrup

- Antibiotics: Cipro (for diarrhea), Bactrim (for UTI), Z-Pack (for upper respiratory infection), Levaquin (for UTIs, skin infection, and severe traveler's diarrhea), Keflex (for insulin pump site infection)
- Contraceptives
- Diamox (for altitude headaches; needs a prescription)
- Famvir (pills for cold sores)
- Tigan suppositories (for nausea and vomiting)
- Sanitary products
- Bee sting kit
- Snake bite kit
- Glucose tablets or glucose gel

OTHER THINGS TO CONSIDER PACKING

You don't need to pack an entire sewing kit, but a few items to get you through in a pinch are helpful: thread in light and dark colors, a needle, a few straight pins, a few safety pins, and several buttons. Some larger hotels provide a small sewing kit for their guests. Remember to pack any sharp, non-essential items in your checked luggage.

Other items you might consider packing include a hair dryer, an iron, or a small hot water pot. To avoid having to carry these appliances with you, you could call ahead or check your hotel's website to see what is provided in your room. Most hotels provide all of these appliances at no extra charge. Many hotels also have coffeepots in the rooms, which you can use to boil water for drinks, dried soups, or snacks. If you are going overseas, you may need to take plug adapters and a transformer, so you can plug your appliances into the direct electric current used there. Your trip will go more smoothly if

you do a little homework before you go
and know what to expect when you get
there.

BE SURE TO PACK HEALTHY FEET

Which shoes and socks?

People with diabetes must take very good
care of their feet. The best way to do this
at home or on a trip is to wear comfortable, well-made shoes that support your
feet, such as running or walking shoes of
leather or a breathable material. On a trip,
you should take several pairs of shoes, so
that you can change them during the day
and prevent blisters from developing.

No matter where you travel, your clothing
should be comfortable and appropriate
for the climate. The most important
items of clothing are your shoes and
socks. Do not buy new shoes and socks
for your trip unless you purchase them
2–3 weeks in advance and have an opportunity to wear them daily to ensure they
fit you properly. It is important to
remember to wear new shoes for only 2–4
hours a day when you are breaking them

Diabetes and Neuropathy

Neuropathy is a long-term complication of diabetes. It is damage to nerves, most often in the feet. Complicating matters, many people with diabetes also have cardiovascular or heart changes that may interfere with the flow of blood to the feet. In the early stages of neuropathy, your feet may be painful, and this pain may get worse over time. Often the pain is most noticeable during the night. As neuropathy progresses, the pain may go away, but it is replaced with a numbness or lack of feeling. When the numbness occurs, there may be little sensation in your feet. At this stage you will not be able to feel a sore, cut, or blister on your feet. You should be careful to wear shoes that fit you well, with no rips or tears in the lining or nails poking through the sole.

in. The shoes you take along should be well broken in and comfortable. They should fit your feet and not cause blisters or calluses.

When you purchase new shoes, be sure there is space the width of your thumb from the end of your longest toe to the end of the shoe. There should be some "give" across the top of the shoe at the widest part of your foot. Your toes should have wiggle room. The heel of the shoe should fit snugly enough, so it does not rub up and down against your heel. It is best if the shoe has an arch support. Look for a shoe with a flexible sole. This will help cushion your foot.

Wear socks that cushion your feet, too. Cushioning in newer socks, such as cotton-acrylic blends, will wick perspiration away from your feet. This is good because perspiration or any moisture on your feet or between your toes may cause your skin to break down, and you could get an infection. However, be sure your socks are not too thick for your shoes and do not have thick seams that press on your toes. You should be able to move your toes inside your shoes with the socks on. If your socks are the correct thickness, your shoes fit comfortably and do not feel too

On the Web

www.medicool.com

This online diabetes supply retailer has hundreds of great products, including shoes, socks, and other foot care products specifically designed for people with diabetes.

tight. There are many socks designed just for people with diabetes. These socks have no seams to irritate your toes and no elastic to cut or pinch feet, and they are made of breathable fabrics.

A journey of a thousand miles starts with one step

Inspecting your feet every day will be even more important when you are traveling and sightseeing. Each morning and again in the evening, look at your feet for reddened areas, blisters, cuts, scratches, sores, or any other changes. If you need a mirror to see the bottom of your feet, be sure to pack one. Be sure to check between your toes. If you need help, don't hesitate to ask a traveling companion (who will cer-

Foot+Saver

You can use a device called the Foot+Saver to look at the bottoms of your feet. The Foot+Saver is a mirror attached to the end of a lightweight aluminum pole with a molded grip. The handle is adjustable, and it swivels and telescopes to make it easier for you to look at all parts of your feet.

1-877-379-2638 or *www.foot-saver.net*

tainly be affected, too, if you develop foot problems).

It is important to follow a basic routine that can prevent foot infections and other complications from happening. The following list of suggestions will help you keep your feet healthy at all times, at home and away from home.

- Inspect your feet every day for blisters, cuts, scratches, or reddened areas.

- Always check between your toes.

- Wash your feet daily. Dry carefully, especially between the toes.

- When you are bathing, avoid extreme temperatures. People who have diabetes may have neuropathy or nerve damage to their feet (see the box *Diabetes and Neuropathy*). You may not be able to determine just how hot the water is. Test the water with your elbow (or a bath thermometer) before bathing. This will prevent you from getting burned.

- If your feet feel cold at night, wear socks. Do not apply a hot water bottle, electric blanket, or heating pad.

- Do not walk on hot surfaces, such as sandy beaches or on the cement around swimming pools. If you must walk in these areas, be sure to wear shoes with a thick enough sole to protect your feet from getting burned.

- Do not use cold packs on your foot or ankle unless instructed to do so by your health care provider.

- Do not walk barefoot anywhere, ever.

- Inspect the inside of your shoes daily for foreign objects, nail points, torn lining, and rough areas.

- Do not soak your feet unless specifically instructed to do so.

- Apply a thin coat of a moisturizing cream daily after bathing. Do not put cream between your toes.

- Wear properly fitting socks. Do not wear mended socks. Avoid socks with thick seams. Change socks daily. Do not wear garters or anything tight around your legs or feet.

- Shoes should be comfortable at the time you buy them. Purchase shoes in the afternoon when feet tend to be the largest. Do not depend on the shoes to stretch to fit you.

- Do not wear shoes without socks or stockings.

- Do not wear sandals with thongs between the toes.

- Cut nails straight across or follow the curve of the nail. If nails are thick or difficult to cut, have a health care provider or podiatrist cut them. Don't risk injuring your foot.

- Do not smoke. Smoking affects the circulation to your legs and feet.

- Do not treat corns or calluses on your own. Consult a health care provider.

On the Web

www.ndep.nih.gov

This is the website for Department of Diabetes Education Programs and it contains information on foot care for people with diabetes, as well as a brochure titled, Feet Can Last a Lifetime. If you don't have access to the internet, you can have the brochure mailed to you by calling 1-800-438-5383 and using NDEP-4 for English and NDEP-48 for Spanish.

Medicare's Therapeutic Shoe Bill

For more information on Medicare's Therapeutic Shoe Bill, visit *www.medicalresourceslimited.com* and click on "Therapeutic Shoe Bill" or call 1-800-998-4199.

For Medicare to pay for your therapeutic shoes, you must have one or more of the following:

a. Neuropathy in your feet and calluses

b. History of calluses leading to ulcers

c. Significant foot deformity

d. Previous amputation of a foot or part of a foot

e. Limited circulation

What types of shoes are covered?

a. Custom-molded shoes

b. Extra-depth shoes

c. Inserts

d. Shoe modifications

Coverage is limited to the following in one calendar year:

a. One pair of custom-molded shoes with inserts and two additional pairs of inserts or,

b. One pair of extra-depth shoes and three pairs of inserts.

c. Modifications of shoes can be substituted for a pair of inserts.

Who provides therapeutic shoes?

Shoes must be fitted and provided by a podiatrist, orthotist, pedorthist, or prosthetist. These professionals must be registered with Medicare. They will fill out the appropriate prescription after your physician has completed the Certification statement.

What is the Certification statement?

The physician who treats your diabetes must certify your need for special shoes.

What are the rules for reimbursement?

The shoe supplier will file the appropriate claim with Medicare. Reimbursement is limited to 80% of the reasonable charge, and there's a maximum amount that Medicare will reimburse.

Do other insurance companies cover therapeutic shoes?

Many other health insurance companies will also reimburse for therapeutic shoes. You will need a prescription from your health care provider. Check with your insurance company regarding the coverage they will provide. Your insurance company will also tell you where you can go to be fitted for therapeutic shoes.

- Never use any medication on your feet without first discussing it with your health care provider.

- If any changes occur to your feet, get in touch with your health care provider immediately.

Before you go, be aware of the shape your feet are in

In later stages of neuropathy, the structure or shape of your foot may change. The muscles that support the bones in your feet are affected by neuropathy. They may allow the bones in your feet to move, and so your feet change shape. Your feet are also more prone to injury. You might notice that your toes begin to curl under and you walk on the tips of your toes rather than the bottom surface of your feet. The arch of your foot may become flat or more pronounced. Bunions may form. All of these changes put stress on the surface skin of your feet. The stressed areas are where calluses develop, and those areas are most at risk for foot ulcers. See your health care provider to discuss the shape your feet are in if you have calluses or your shoes no longer fit well.

If you have neuropathy and changes in the structure of your feet, talk with your provider about getting therapeutic shoes or inserts. These shoes are specially fitted to your feet so they can protect your feet from developing ulcers. Your health insurance may cover some or all of the cost of these specially made shoes (see the box *Medicare's Therapeutic Shoe Bill*). The newer types of therapeutic shoes are more attractive. Some shoes have a larger toe box so your toes will fit comfortably and your feet are protected. Allow enough time to get these shoes, and wear them for several weeks before traveling to be sure they fit you comfortably.

Chapter Three

INSULIN, SYMLIN, BYETTA & YOUR TRAVELS

All people with type 1 diabetes need to take insulin injections. About 40% of people with type 2 diabetes also take insulin. As you well know, it can be tricky trying to time insulin action with the digestion of your meals to keep blood glucose near normal levels. So, following a familiar schedule of meals, snacks, exercise, and injections can help your trip go more smoothly. But so many things can affect your blood glucose level: if you miss a meal or get much more exercise than usual, or you're in a different time zone, or you get ill. And the stress that you feel having to cope with new situations affects your blood glucose, too! So, be flexible and use the information in this book to help you keep your balance.

Being organized is the key to smooth sailing and successful travel. Any change of routine—traveling, staying in a hotel, visiting someone else's home—can make you forget to take your insulin. If you have everything with you in your bag or cooler, you're more likely to remember to use it.

IN YOUR CARRY-ON BAG

When you pack your insulin, Symlin, Byetta, syringes, blood glucose meter, test strips, ketone strips, and glucagon kit, pack twice as many supplies as you think you will need. Keep them with you throughout the trip. Never put them in your checked baggage in case they get lost or damaged en route. If security situations prohibit carry-on luggage, provide proof to security that you have diabetes and must have your carry-on bag and insulin with you at all times. Also carry glucose products (see the box *Over-the-Counter Products to Treat Low Blood Glucose*)

Over-the-Counter Products to Treat Low Blood Glucose

Product Name/Manufacturer	Carbohydrate/Dose	Calories	Form
B-D Glucose Tablets (Becton Dickinson)	5 g/tablet	20	Orange flavored tablets
Dex4 Glucose Tablets (Can-Am Care)	4 g/tablet	15	Orange, watermelon, raspberry, or grape flavored tablets
Glutose 45 (3 dose) (Paddock Laboratories)	15 g/dose (3-dose resealable tube)	60/dose	Natural lemon flavored gel
Glutose 15 (Paddock Laboratories)	15 g/dose (1 dose/tube)	60	Natural lemon flavored gel
Insta-Glucose (Valeant Pharmaceuticals, Inc.)	24 g/1 dose tube	96	Cherry flavored gel
Various store brand glucose tablets	4 g/tablet	15	10-count tubes and 50-count bottles. Flavors: apple, cherry, coconut, assorted fruit and strawberry cream quick dissolve.

Adapted from *The Diabetes Forecast Resource Guide*, 2006.

and foods to treat low blood glucose and snacks for 24 hours. All of this might make your tote bag a little heavy at the start of the trip, but these items will keep you healthy and relieve you of worry time and again.

If you haven't already, discuss how to use a glucagon kit to treat a serious low blood glucose level with your health care provider (see the box *Glucagon*). Be sure that at least one person traveling with you knows that you have diabetes and how to treat your low blood glucose, including how to use the glucagon if necessary.

One more thing about snacks

If you take insulin, you must have snacks or glucose products with you all the time. You should never risk having low blood glucose anywhere you go. At your destination when you are walking all day sightseeing, you are likely to get more exercise than usual. You'll need an extra snack between meals, preferably protein and carbohydrate, such as cheese and crackers or half a meat sandwich. Children with diabetes need snacks throughout the day and

Glucagon

If you take insulin or other medications that can cause low blood glucose, you need a glucagon kit. Glucagon, when injected into the body, stimulates the liver to release stored glucose and is used in emergency situations when glucose is severely low, oral treatments are not working quickly enough, or the person with low blood glucose is unconscious or unable to take oral treatments. Have your doctor train you and your loved ones on how to administer glucagon. Following is a basic explanation.

1. A glucagon kit has a syringe filled with diluting fluid and a bottle of powdered glucagon. The person helping you must mix the diluting fluid with the powder before it can be injected. The instructions for mixing and injecting glucagon are included in the kit.

2. Inject glucagon in the same way and in the same parts of the body that people inject insulin. It may also be given into a muscle.

3. If glucagon is mixed in a syringe but not used, you may refrigerate the capped syringe and store it for up to 2 days. Contact the manufacturer for more details.

4. The person with low blood glucose should respond to the glucagon injection in 15–30 minutes. If he or she does not respond, call emergency personnel (911 in the U.S.).

5. After the injection, nausea and vomiting are common. Keep the person getting the injection turned to the side.

6. As soon as the person can swallow, offer regular soda, crackers, or toast.

7. Then offer a sandwich or protein snack.

8. Check blood glucose.

at bedtime, too. On airplanes or at restaurants, they may not like the food available. You might not either. Pack items that you and they will eat to keep on schedule and to prevent low blood glucose. In fact, it will be wise to pack a small suitcase with a variety of snacks. You might start with the list of snacks in the box *Travel Snacks to Carry* on page 28.

You can use glucose tablets, gels, or liquid to treat low blood glucose (see the box *Over-the-Counter Products to Treat Low Blood Glucose*). They are easy to carry, but try them out before you travel. You may not care for the taste or consistency of one of the products.

Your prescription letter

You should also carry with you a prescription or letter from your health care provider with information about the insulin and syringes you use and all other injectable medication you may be taking (see the *Example of a Prescription Letter* on page 10). The letter should state (and you should know) the types of medication you use, the concentration (Table 3-1), the dose(s), and the size and gauge of your insulin syringe.

INSULIN RULES OF THE ROAD

Insulin in opened bottles is safe for about 1 month if you keep it at normal room temperature. It should not get hotter than 86 degrees or colder than 40 degrees. To remember when you opened the bottle, write the date on the label.

How to store insulin, Symlin, and Byetta

Manufacturers of insulin recommend that you store it in the refrigerator. This is to protect it from extreme changes in temperature, which can affect its potency. However, injecting cold insulin can make injections uncomfortable. It is also difficult to keep insulin in a refrigerator when you're on the road. Insulin can be kept at room temperature for 30 days.

The guidelines for storing prefilled insulin pens and insulin cartridges are different. Regular and lispro (Humalog) prefilled pens and cartridges can be used

Table 3-1. Insulins Commonly

Generic Name	Brand Names
RAPID-ACTING	
insulin lispro	Humalog
insulin aspart	NovoLog
insulin glulisine	Apidra
REGULAR	
regular	Humulin R
regular	Novolin R, ReliOn (Wal-Mart)
INTERMEDIATE-ACTING	
NPH	Humulin N
NPH	Novolin N, ReliOn (Wal-Mart)
LONG-ACTING	
insulin glargine	Lantus
insulin detemir	Levemir
MIXTURES	
70% NPH/30% regular	Humulin 70/30
70% NPH/30% regular	Novolin 70/30, ReliOn (Wal-Mart)
75% lispro protamine/ (NPL) 25% lispro	Humalog Mix 75/25
70% aspart protamine/ 30% aspart	NovoLog Mix 70/30

Used in the United States

Form	Manufacturer	Cloudy/Clear
analog	Eli Lilly and Company	clear
analog	Novo Nordisk, Inc.	clear
analog	sanofi aventis	clear
human	Eli Lilly and Company	clear
human	Novo Nordisk, Inc.	clear
human	Eli Lilly and Company	cloudy
human	Novo Nordisk, Inc.	cloudy
analog	sanofi aventis	clear
analog	Novo Nordisk, Inc.	clear
human	Eli Lilly and Company	cloudy
human	Novo Nordisk, Inc.	cloudy
analog	Eli Lilly and Company	cloudy
analog	Novo Nordisk, Inc.	cloudy

Adapted from *The Diabetes Forecast Resource Guide*, 2006

at room temperature for up to 30 days after first use. Prefilled pens containing NPH and 70/30 can be stored at room temperature for 7 days after first use. Pens with 75/25 can be stored 10 days. Keeping your insulin in a cooler or cool pack can protect it from temperature extremes and from being knocked around in a purse or backpack.

The manufacturers of Symlin recommend that you store unopened vials in the refrigerator. Open vials may be kept either in the refrigerator or at room temperature. However, it is best to inject Symlin at room temperature. After a vial is open, it can be used for up to 28 days.

Byetta should be kept refrigerated. Each pen contains enough medication for 30 days of two injections each day. Once you start to use a Byetta pen, it can only be kept at room temperature for a total of 6 days after initial use. It is best to keep the pen in either a refrigerator or cool pack.

If you will be on the go all day and plan to keep your insulin, Symlin, or Byetta with you, then purchasing a cool pack

Symlin and Byetta

Symlin (pramlintide injectable)

Symlin is a synthetic version of the hormone amylin. Symlin improves blood glucose control by working with insulin in three ways. It:

1. Helps food move out of the stomach at a slower rate.

2. Reduces the amount of glucose the liver sends into the bloodstream after meals.

3. Regulates food intake by decreasing appetite.

Byetta (exenatide)

Byetta works with diabetes pills to help the body produce the right amount of insulin. Byetta works in four ways:

1. It signals the pancreas to make the correct amount of insulin at meals. Once blood glucose levels get closer to normal, Byetta stops causing the pancreas to produce more insulin.

2. Byetta helps stop the liver from producing too much sugar when the body doesn't need it.

3. Byetta helps slow down the rate at which sugar enters your bloodstream.

4. Byetta has been shown to reduce food intake.

(see the box *Carrying Cases with an Insulin Cool Pack*) is in order. This may be the most important carry-on bag you ever own. If you will take your insulin in the morning before you leave the hotel and again when you return in the evening, you may be able to keep it in a refrigerator in your hotel room. Be sure to check that the hotel or other place at which you are staying does indeed have a refrigerator.

Never leave injectable medication in a car. In warm weather, the car will be too warm for the insulin, Symlin, and Byetta, and in cold weather, the car will be too cold. Do not pack insulin, Symlin, or Byetta in a suitcase that will be checked at an airport. The baggage compartment is not climate controlled.

> ! Do not pack your insulin, Symlin, or
> Byetta in checked luggage. Keep it with
> • you in your carry-on bag at all times.

Some one-day tourist destinations, such as amusement parks or water parks, will often store your injectable medication in the refrigerator at the first aid station. Call ahead to check before you get to the

Carrying Cases with an Insulin Cool Pack

These cases can help you organize your diabetes supplies. They vary in size and will fit specific needs.

- **Apothecary Products**
  Insulated Diabetic Wallet
  www.apothecaryproducts.com

- **Frio Cooling Products**
  FRIO Wallets (As opposed to freezing, the FRIO pack is run under cold water for 5-7 minutes. The gel pack will then keep medications cool for 3-5 days. It is also reuseable.)
  www.wisechoicefrio.com

- **Medicool, Inc.**
  Dia-Pak Classic, Deluxe, and Daymate
  Insulin Protector
  ProtectAll Pack
  www.medicool.com

- **MEDport**
  The Wallet Organizer
  The Daily Organizer
  The Travel Organizer
  MEDport Replacement Ice Pack
  www.medportllc.com

park. While this can make for less to lug around, it's still a better idea to keep your injectable medication with you in a protected cool pack.

Make a habit of inspecting your insulin and other injectable medication for damage or loss of potency each time you use it. Are there any changes in appearance? Is it discolored? Are there any large particles present in the liquid? Are there salt- or sugar-like crystals gathered on the narrowed portion of the vial? Has your medication that is supposed to be clear become cloudy? If any of these changes have occurred, the vial or cartridge should be thrown away. Other changes to the potency are not visible, so be alert for signs that your injectable medication is not lowering your blood glucose as it should, especially when there is no other explanation. This is true of insulin for a pump as well. Always date your insulin, Symlin, or Byetta when you open it, store it correctly, and throw it away after 4 weeks or whenever the manufacturer recommends.

TRASH IS IMPORTANT

When you're on the road, be sure to dispose of your used syringes, pen needles, insulin pump infusion needle and lines, and lancets safely. Carelessly leaving them in trashcans at hotels or restaurants can frighten and endanger other people, and it is illegal. You may purchase a personal-size safety disposal box. It is small enough to fit in your carry-on bag or suitcase. At the end of your trip, it can be disposed of at home in accordance with the regulations in your area.

Needle Clipper

When traveling, you might consider a needle clipper, such as the BD Safe-Clip, which can be purchased in most drug stores. A needle clipper is a small device that clips off the needle of your syringe and automatically stores the needle tip. Although the device is very small, it will store up to 2 years of needle tips, and when full, you can dispose of the entire device. The rest of the syringe can be thrown away in the regular trash. This device eliminates the need to carry around syringes until you can safely dispose of them.

Reusing Syringes for Insulin

1. Carefully recap the syringe when you aren't using it.

2. Don't let the needle touch anything but clean skin and your insulin bottle stopper. If it touches anything else, don't reuse it.

3. Store used syringes at room temperature.

4. There will always be a tiny, even invisible, amount of insulin left in the syringe. So use one syringe with just one type of insulin to avoid mixing insulins or contaminating the vials. For this reason, reusing syringes in which you have mixed insulins is not recommended.

5. Do not reuse a needle that is bent or dull. However, just because an injection is painful, doesn't mean the needle is dull. You may have hit a nerve ending or have wet alcohol on your skin (if you cleaned the injection site with alcohol).

6. Do not wipe your needle with alcohol. This removes some of the coating that makes the needle go more smoothly into your skin.

7. When you're finished with a syringe, dispose of it properly according to the laws in your area. Contact the city or county sanitation department for information.

You can reuse your insulin syringes, pen needles for insulin, and lancets (see the box *Reusing Syringes for Insulin*). However, it is not recommended that you reuse insulin syringes or pen needles for either Symlin or Byetta. Even if you choose not to reuse them when you are home, you may want to reuse syringes for insulin when you travel to cut down on how much you have to carry with you.

CHECK FOR KETONES

Even if you do not use them at home, you need to carry ketone test strips with you while you travel. If you get ill or if your blood glucose goes higher than 250 mg/dl, it is very important for you to check your urine for ketones (see the box *Ketone Testing*). It will also allow a health care provider to better guide you in your care if you have both blood glucose and ketone values.

Ketones in your urine are a warning sign that your body is burning fat for fuel rather than glucose. This could mean that your diabetes is out of control. If you have ketones in your urine, you may need extra insulin. People who have type 2 diabetes do not usually produce ketones in their urine, but if you have type 2 diabetes and become ill, it's a good idea to check your urine for ketones anyway. It's the sign of a serious condition developing. Whether you have type 1 or type 2 diabetes, if you

Ketone Testing

If your blood glucose is 250 mg/dl or higher and it cannot be explained by what you have just eaten, check for ketones in your urine.

Equipment:
- Ketone test strip
- Cup or clean container for sample
- A watch or other timing device

1. Dip a ketone test strip in a urine sample or pass it through the stream of urine.
2. Time the test according to the directions on the package.
3. The strip will change colors if ketones are present. Compare the test strip to the color chart on the package.
4. Record the results and have them available when you call your health care provider for guidance.

have ketones in your urine, contact a health care provider right away.

Several companies now make a blood glucose meter that uses two types of blood glucose test strips. One test strip is designed to monitor blood for glucose. The second test strip is used to check blood for ketones. You may prefer to use this method of testing for ketones as opposed to the urine strips.

WATCH OUT! THE INSULIN AND SYRINGES ARE FOREIGN, TOO

Insulin

Be aware that the names of insulin may be different in other countries. For example, the 70/30 mixture you use may be called 30/70 there. Read the labels very carefully. If you are using a newer insulin or other injectable medication, it may not be available outside the United States. You may wish to contact the manufacturer directly and ask. If the medication is available, find out what it is called in the country to which you will be traveling. Many manufacturers also have websites you can visit online for information and assistance.

The concentration of insulin in the United States is U-100. This means that you get 100 units of insulin in 1 ml of fluid. In Europe and other countries, the concentration of insulin is usually U-40. This means that you get 40 units of insulin in 1 ml of fluid. If, somehow, you have to use U-40 insulin, be sure you also use a U-40 insulin syringe and not the syringes you brought with you. If your usual dose is 20 units of U-100 insulin, your dose will be the same with U-40 insulin as long as you use a U-40 insulin syringe. You will still take 20 units of insulin, you will just be injecting more fluid.

> ! If you need to take U-40 insulin, use a U-40 syringe. Otherwise, you will need to recalculate your dose.

If you use a U-100 syringe with U-40 insulin and do not adjust the dose, you will be taking less than 1/2 of your usual dose of insulin. You need to take 2 1/2 times as much U-40 insulin to get your

Diabetes Survival Kit

Put in your survival kit the things that you want to have with you on your travels. Some of them you may already be carrying with you every time you go out the door. Use this checklist to help you start creating your own survival kit.

- Insulin supplies:
  - insulin, syringes, disposal case
  - letter/prescription with your doses and types of insulin
- Extra prescriptions for diabetes medications and supplies
- Note from doctor about your need for diabetes supplies
- Insulated travel bag for insulin and other injectable medications that need refrigeration
- Medications
- Glucagon kit
- Glucose tablets or quick-acting low blood glucose treatment
- Meter and test strips
- Extra batteries
- Extra meter
- Lancing device, lancets
- Extra lancing device
- Written directions on how to take your insulin
- Phone numbers of your health care team
- Medical ID stating that you have diabetes
- Insulin pens
- Pump supplies
- Urine ketone strips
- Snacks (at least twice as many as you think you need)
- Sick-day insulin program
- Off pump–day program
- Notebook and pen
- Moist towelettes
- Hand cream

proper dose. For example, if you usually take 10 units of U-100 insulin, but need to use U-40 insulin with a U-100 syringe, multiply by 2 1/2 to get your new dose.

10 units × 2.5 = 25 units of insulin

If you're using U-100 insulin in a U-40 syringe, you'd do the opposite; divide by 2 1/2. In situations where insulin and syringes don't match, ask a local health professional to help you make the conversion.

Syringes

Syringes are available in different sizes. The common insulin syringes hold 30, 50, or 100 units of insulin. The length and diameter of the needle also varies. If you must use a syringe that is different from your usual one, look to see whether the numbers on the side of the syringe are in 1/2-unit, 1-unit, or 2-unit increments. If the numbers are even numbers (2, 4, 6), then the syringe measures 2 units of insulin. If the numbers are odd numbers (1, 3, 5), then it measures 1-unit increments. You need to know so you can draw up the correct amount of insulin.

Insulin pens

Insulin pens were used overseas long before they were used in the United States. If you are presently using insulin pens, you should not have any difficulty finding supplies if you need them.

CROSSING TIME ZONES

If you are traveling to a different time zone, you will have to make adjustments to the time you take your insulin, Symlin, or Byetta. It is important to adjust your schedule to the new time zone as quickly as possible.

Adjusting insulin

Usually if the time change is less than 3 hours, taking your injectable medication based on the new time will be fine. If the time change is 3 hours or more, then you must make some changes in the timing of your medication to make the transition to the new time zone as smooth as possible. You'll also make adjustments in your program on the way home, as you return to your usual time zone. The following sections about injectable medication adjustments are suggestions, not rules. Discuss how much to adjust your medication with your health care provider.

Adjusting insulin for one or two time zone changes

The time change is 1 or 2 hours and you take one or more insulin injections per day. On the day of travel, take your insulin based on your home time. Begin using the local time in the morning of the first full day at your destination.

Traveling east

You have a time change of 3 or more hours to the east (travel day shortened).

Adjusting for one injection a day

On your travel day, you may take your insulin as you usually do or decrease it by 10–20%. On the first full day at your destination, wake on the local time schedule and take your usual dose of insulin. Continue to take your insulin at the same time each day using the local time.

Adjusting for two or more injections a day

On your travel day, decrease the last daily dose of intermediate- or long-acting insulin by 20%. On the first full day at your destination, wake on the local time schedule and take your usual dose of insulin. Continue to take your insulin based on the local time.

For example:

Home 20 units NPH, 10 units rapid-acting before breakfast, 10 units rapid-acting before lunch

    20 units NPH, 10 units rapid-acting before dinner

Travel 20 units NPH, 10 units rapid-acting before breakfast on home time

    10 units rapid-acting before lunch, taken on home time

    16 units NPH, 10 units rapid-acting before dinner on home time

Destination   20 units NPH, 10 units rapid-acting before breakfast on destination time

10 units rapid-acting before lunch on destination time

20 units NPH, 10 units rapid-acting before dinner on destination time

Traveling west

You have a time change of 3 or more hours to the west (travel day lengthened).

Adjusting for one injection a day

On your travel day, take your insulin as you usually do. Since the day will be longer, you may need a second injection of insulin in the early evening. If you take only intermediate-acting insulin at breakfast, you may need a second injection of the same insulin before dinner. The injection time should be based on your home time, not your destination time. The dose should be 1/3 of your morning dose.

For example:

Home   60 units NPH at breakfast
                on home time

Travel   60 units NPH at breakfast

                20 units NPH before din-
                ner on home time

Destination 60 units NPH at breakfast
                on local time

If your morning injection is a combination of intermediate- and rapid-acting
insulin, then your second injection should
be the same combination. The time of the
dose should be before dinner based on
your home time not your destination
time. The dose should be 1/3 of your
morning dose.

For example:

Home   40 units NPH, 20 units
                rapid-acting at breakfast
                on home time

Travel   40 units NPH, 20 units
                rapid-acting at breakfast

12 units NPH, 7 units
rapid-acting before dinner
on home time

Destination 40 units NPH, 20 units
rapid-acting on local time

If your morning injection is an insulin
mix of 70/30, 75/25, or 50/50, take your
morning injection based on your home
time. Your second injection should be 1/3
of your breakfast injection taken before
dinner based on your home time.

For example:

Home 50 units 70/30 at breakfast
on home time

Travel 50 units 70/30 at breakfast

15 units 70/30 before dinner on home time

Destination 50 units 70/30 at breakfast
on local time

Another option would be to take your
usual morning injection based on your
home time. If you eat an extra meal, take

an injection of rapid-acting insulin to cover the carbohydrate content of the meal. As a rule of thumb, 1 unit of rapid-acting insulin covers 15 g of carbohydrate. (But this varies by individual, so be sure to check your blood glucose to see how you respond to carbohydrate. If you know your personal ratio for insulin-to-carb, use it.)

For example:

Home	60 units NPH at breakfast on home time
Travel	60 units NPH at breakfast
	4 units rapid-acting insulin at dinner (meal with 60 g carbohydrate)
Destination	60 units NPH at breakfast on local time

Adjusting for two or more injections a day

On your travel day, take your breakfast insulin as you usually do based on your home time schedule. If you take insulin at lunchtime, take your usual dose based on your home time schedule. Take your usual dinnertime rapid-acting insulin at your dinner meal. If your last daily injection of intermediate- or long-acting insulin is usually at dinnertime, delay it 3 hours and decrease the dose by 20%.

For example:

Home	20 units NPH, 10 units rapid-acting before breakfast
	20 units NPH, 10 units rapid-acting before dinner
Travel	20 units NPH, 10 units rapid-acting before breakfast on home time
	10 units rapid-acting before dinner is served
	16 units NPH at 9–10 PM based on destination time
Destination	Wake on destination time and take 20 units NPH

10 units rapid-acting before breakfast

20 units NPH, 10 units rapid-acting before dinner

Example including insulin taken before lunch:

Home   20 units NPH, 10 units rapid-acting before breakfast

10 units rapid-acting before lunch

20 units NPH, 10 units rapid-acting before dinner

Travel   20 units NPH, 10 units rapid-acting before break-fast on home time

10 units rapid-acting before lunch is served

10 units rapid-acting before dinner is served

16 units NPH at 9–10 PM based on destination time

Destination   Wake on destination time
and take 20 units NPH

10 units rapid-acting
before breakfast

10 units rapid-acting
before lunch

20 units NPH, 10 units
rapid-acting before dinner

If your last daily injection of intermediate-
or long-acting insulin is usually at
9:00–10:00 PM, take this injection at the
same time you would based on your home
time and increase this dose by 10%.

For example:

Home   20 units NPH, 10 units
rapid-acting before
breakfast

10 units rapid-acting
before lunch

10 units rapid-acting
before dinner

20 units NPH at 9–10 PM

Travel	20 units NPH, 10 units rapid-acting before breakfast on home time
	10 units rapid-acting before lunch is served
	10 units rapid-acting before dinner is served
	22 units NPH at 9–10 PM based on home time
Destination	Wake on destination time, 20 units NPH
	10 units rapid-acting before breakfast
	10 units rapid-acting before lunch
	10 units rapid-acting before dinner
	20 units NPH at 9–10 PM

When you arrive at your destination, wake on the destination time and take your usual insulin doses based on your destination time schedule. Discuss with your health care professional what to do if an extra meal is served. It is possible that you can cover the carbohydrate content of the meal using 1 unit of rapid-acting insulin for each 15 g of carbohydrate or one starch, fruit, or milk serving. (Again, this varies by individual.)

If you take a long-acting insulin at bed (9:00–10:00 PM) and rapid-acting insulin before each meal, use the information for NPH at breakfast and 9:00–10:00 PM, omitting the breakfast NPH.

Adjusting Symlin and Byetta for Travel

Symlin

Since Symlin is taken with meals, Symlin should be taken with rapid-acting insulin after insulin adjustments for travel are made.

Byetta

Byetta is taken twice daily with meals. Injections should be approximately 8–10 hours apart. When you arrive at your destination, get onto the new time zone as quickly as possible and continue to take the Byetta with the meals you usually do. Be sure your first injection at your new destination is at least 8–10 hours after the last injection of Byetta you took while traveling.

Adjusting your pump for time zones

Set the insulin pump clock to the destination time zone at any time during your
flight. Set your basal rate to a constant
daytime basal rate over the 24-hour schedule for the pump while traveling. Measure
your blood glucose several times during
the trip. Bolus to cover snacks, meals, and
elevated blood glucose levels. When you
arrive at your destination, reset your multiple basal rates based on your blood glucose readings and the destination time
zone.

TRAVELING WITH AN INSULIN PUMP

If you wear an insulin pump, pack extra
pump supplies, carry the toll-free phone
number of your insulin pump company,
and pack a vial of long-acting
(Lantus/Detimir SP) or intermediate-acting (NPH/lente) insulin just in case. If
your pump breaks down, most insulin
pump companies are able to ship an
insulin pump to you within 24 hours as
long as the pump is under warranty. If the

pump is not still under warranty, but your insurance company will purchase a new pump for you, you can usually get a new one in several days with the assistance of your health care provider. (This is why you need to take extra insulin with you to use until you get the new pump.) The pump manufacturer will usually agree to ship you a loaner pump within 24 hours while the paperwork is being completed and approval is obtained from your insurance company. If your pump is out of warranty and your insurance company won't pay for a new pump, you may purchase a pump at your own expense.

Most insulin pumps have a warranty of around 4 years and most insurance companies will purchase a new insulin pump if you need one—every 4-6 years. It is a good idea to know the length and extent of the warranty on your insulin pump. You should also know the benefits your insurance company will provide and how often you can get a new insulin pump.

If you need to use a loaner pump, try to get the same model you are currently using. If this is not possible, be sure to review the owner's manual, manufacturer's website, or call the customer help line to assist you before you start using your new loaner pump. If you end up purchasing a new pump, it will definitely have new features, so learn the basics as best you can. Make an appointment to visit your health care provider as soon as you return home to learn more about how to use your new pump. Whether you get a loaner pump or a new pump, it will not be set with your basal rates or bolus rations. Be sure to write down your rates to carry with you and program that information in before you start using the pump.

In the meantime, while the details are being worked out, you will need to take insulin by syringe or insulin pen. Some people prefer to use just rapid-acting insulin in multiple injections until a new pump arrives. Others prefer to use an injection of long- or intermediate-acting insulin at bedtime and then multiple injections of rapid-acting insulin during the day. If the pump will not arrive for several days, and you choose to use intermediate-acting insulin, you may wish to

take intermediate-acting insulin at breakfast and bedtime and rapid-acting insulin
before each meal. You may already have a
plan that you use for the days when you
do not wear your pump. If you do not
have a plan, be sure to discuss this with
your health care team before you travel. It
is best if you have a plan written down
and keep it with your important travel
papers.

> If you don't have a plan for going off
> the pump, develop one with your
> health care provider before leaving.

Taking time off your insulin pump

If you remove your insulin pump for a few
hours, check your blood glucose several
times to see whether you will need to take
any insulin by insulin pen or injection.
Often, if you've been physically active,
you may not need to. If your blood glucose level rises while you're off your
pump, you may calculate how long you
have been off the pump, determine how
much basal rate of insulin you have
missed, and take that amount by insulin
syringe or insulin pen.

For example, you remove your insulin pump from 2:00 PM until 4:30 PM. Your blood glucose at 4:30 PM is 180 mg/dl. Your usual basal rate from 2:00 PM until 4:30 PM is 0.8 units per hour. You have not received 2 units of basal insulin while you were off your insulin pump.

$$\begin{array}{r} \text{2 1/2 hours off your pump} \\ \times\ \text{0.8 units per hour} \\ \hline = \text{2 units of insulin} \end{array}$$

Take 2 units of rapid-acting or regular insulin by syringe or insulin pen, or if you will be hooking up your pump at this time, bolus 2 units of insulin.

Another way to figure how much insulin you need: Allow 1 unit of insulin for each 25 mg/dl you wish to lower your blood glucose. If your blood glucose is 200 mg/dl and you wish to lower your blood glucose to 125 mg/dl, you might take 3 units of regular or rapid-acting insulin. But you need to know how quickly you respond to insulin! Some people only need 1 unit of insulin for every 50 mg/dl they wish to lower their blood glucose.

The first time you use this formula, try using 1 unit of insulin for every 50 mg/dl you wish to lower your blood glucose. If this does not get your blood glucose level where you would like it, then try using 1 unit of insulin for every 25 mg/dl you want to lower your blood glucose. If you already have a sensitivty ratio, use it.

If your insulin pump malfunctions and you will be off your insulin pump for 24 hours or more, you will need to take long-acting (Lantus or Detimir) or intermedi-ate-acting (NPH or lente) insulin. To determine how much long- or intermedi-ate-acting insulin you need, add up all of your basal doses for 24 hours. If you will be using long-acting insulin for your basal insulin, take this number of units of insulin at 10:00 PM. If you will be using intermediate-acting insulin, divide this number by 2, because you will take half of your basal rate insulin in the form of intermediate-acting insulin before break-fast and the other half at 10:00 PM. You will continue to take your usual boluses before each meal using rapid-acting insulin with a syringe or insulin pen.

Using intermediate-acting insulin as your basal rate:

Your basal rates are:

Midnight to 3 AM	3.0
3 AM to 6 AM	2.4
6 AM to 10 AM	4.8
10 AM to 9 PM	6.6
9 PM to midnight	2.4

The total daily basal rate of insulin is 19.2 units per 24 hours.

$$19.2 \div 2 = 9.6 \text{ units of insulin}$$

Round 9.6 up to 10, so you know to take 10 units of intermediate-acting insulin before breakfast and 10 units at 10:00 PM.

Your pump breaks down at 5:00 PM on Monday afternoon. Your new pump will arrive on Wednesday by 2:00 PM. Monday night at 10:00 PM you take 10 units of intermediate-acting insulin. Tuesday before breakfast, take 10 units of interme- diate-acting insulin and your usual dose of intermediate-acting insulin. At lunch and dinner, take your usual dose of rapid-acting insulin. At 10:00 PM, take 10 units of intermediate-acting insulin. Wednesday before breakfast, take 10 units of intermediate-acting insulin and your usual dose of rapid-acting insulin. At lunch take your usual dose of rapid-acting insulin. When your insulin pump arrives, be sure to program your basal rates before you attach it. Stop taking the intermediate-acting insulin.

Using long-acting insulin as your basal rate

Your basal rates are:

Midnight to 3 AM	2.4
3 AM to 6 AM	3.0
6 AM to 5 PM	7.7
5 PM to midnight	5.6

The total daily basal insulin is 18.7 units per 24 hours. Round this number to 19 units. You will take 19 units of long-acting insulin at 10:00 PM.

Your pump breaks down at noon on Wednesday. Your new insulin pump will arrive on Friday by 2:00 PM. For lunch and dinner, take your usual bolus of rapid-acting insulin. At 10:00 PM take 19 units of long-acting insulin. Thursday, take your usual bolus of rapid-acting insulin. At 10:00 PM take 19 units of long-acting insulin. Friday, take your usual bolus of rapid-acting insulin before meals. When your insulin pump arrives, program in your basal rates and, if appropriate to the model, your bolus ratio and correction bolus ratio. Stop taking the long-acting insulin.

The new pump

When a new insulin pump arrives, it may not be the same model you were wearing. There may be differences in the way you operate it. Be sure to review how to use the new pump by calling the pump manufacturer's toll-free phone number or visiting their website. They will help you enter your basal rates, learn the bolus function, and understand the basic workings of the new pump, which should be enough until you are back home and can get more training (see the box *Insulin Pump Phone Numbers and Websites*).

Insulin Pump Phone Numbers and Websites

Animas
(Animas IR 1250)
www.animascorp.com
In the U.S.   1-800-767-7373
From outside the U.S.   1.610.644.8990

Insulet Corporation
(OmniPod Insulin Management System)
www.myomnipod.com
Toll-free number   1-800-591-3455

Medtronic Diabetes
(Minimed Paradigm 515, 715)
www.medtronic-diabetes.com
In the U.S.   1-800-646-4633
Australia/New Zealand   +61 1800 777 808
England   +44 (0) 1923 205142

Nipro Diabetes Systems
(Amigo)
www.niprodiabetes.com
Toll-free number   1-888-651-7867

Smiths Medical MD, Inc.
(CozMore Insulin Technology System)
www.cozmore.com
Toll-free number   1-800-826-9703
Canada   1-866-662-6966

Sooil Development
(DANA Diabecare II)
www.sooilusa.com
Toll-free number   1-866-747-6645

Chapter Four

DIABETES PILLS & YOUR TRAVELS

Organization is the key to smooth sailing and successful travel. Any change of routine, such as traveling or staying in a hotel or someone's home, can make you forget to take your diabetes pills. You might not think that's true, but it happens, even when you are at home and someone or something disrupts your daily routine.

If you don't already have one, get one of those plastic pill organizers with sections for the days of the week, so you can tell at a glance whether you have taken your pills. These organizers are lightweight and can be carried with you in your tote bag or backpack for the day. You might look for the newer styles that actually lock so that there is no chance that your pills will spill out during travel. As always, it is very important that you keep all of your medications with you at all times.

It's also important to check your blood glucose, especially when you're under stress or getting more physical activity than usual. Both can have a significant effect on your blood glucose levels.

A MEAL PLAN IS QUITE IMPORTANT

If you have a meal plan and it works pretty well with your medications and exercise, then it will help you a great deal if you can continue to eat the same number of meals and snacks on your trip that you are accustomed to having. (That's a reason to carry some food with you—so you can eat when you usually do.) Also, the meals and snacks should contain about the same amount of carbohydrate as the meals at home. You may have to be creative to fit local dishes into your meal plan, so ask your dietitian for help with this before you leave. Do some research before you go to find the amount of carbohydrate in the foods you will probably find at your destination, because it's carbohydrate that makes blood glucose rise. For instance, one flour tortilla contains 15 g of carbohydrate, just as one slice of bread and 1/3 cup of rice do.

Meal Planning Helpers

To help you with your research, the ADA has several handy books with lists of the nutrients in many foods, including Lea Ann Holzmiester's *The Diabetes Carb & Fat Gram Guide*, Hope Warshaw's *Guide to Healthy Restaurant Eating*, and the *Exchange Lists for Meal Planning*. You can also find this information from books in the library. Or you can go to the ADA's website at *www.diabetes.org* for this information. If you do not have a computer available, try your local library.

Carry food with you

You never know when you might be unable to find something to eat. Or when you might not like the food that is available. Or when the tour bus will break down in the middle of the jungle. Or when your hosts' schedule doesn't match your own. Just in case, you should always have at least one snack with you, such as cheese and crackers, fruit, a nutrition bar, or a small sandwich. You may be the only person on the plane with something to eat! Check pages 26–29 for more snack ideas.

If your diabetes pills can cause you to have low blood glucose, you need to have food or glucose products (see the box *Over-the-Counter Products to Treat Low Blood Glucose* on page 51) with you to raise your glucose level. Find out from your health care provider if this is a concern for you.

A LETTER FROM YOUR PROVIDER

As we discussed in chapter 1, it is important to carry with you a letter from your health care provider stating that you have diabetes, and you need to have your diabetes meter and lancets with you. You also need to bring extra prescriptions for your diabetes pills in case you need to buy

Type 2 Diabetes Survival Kit

Use this list to create your own survival kit. You may want to carry it with you everyday.

- Oral diabetes medications
- Letter giving dosage and directions for when and how to take medications
- Letter from health care provider stating your need for diabetes supplies
- Extra prescriptions for diabetes medications and supplies
- Written directions for how and when to adjust your dosage
- Glucagon kit (if your medication can cause low blood glucose)
- Glucose tablets or other quick-acting treatment for low blood glucose
- Meter, test strips, and battery
- Extra batteries
- Extra meter
- Lancing device
- Extra lancing device
- Phone numbers of your health care team
- Medical ID on you stating that you have diabetes
- Urine ketone strips
- Snacks (about twice as many as you think you need)
- Sick-day program
- Moist towelettes
- Hand cream
- Lip balm
- Notebook and pen

more. You should know which pills you are taking (Table 4-1), but also carry a letter listing the diabetes pills, the dosages, and the times you should take them. The letter might also say whether your medication can cause low blood glucose and what to do about it, in case others need to help you.

CAN YOUR DIABETES PILLS CAUSE LOW BLOOD GLUCOSE?

You need to know the answer to this question. Diabetes medications work in different ways to balance the effect of the food that you eat (Table 4-2). If your diabetes medications (especially if you take several of them) can cause your blood glucose to go too low, then you need to always carry glucose tablets or snacks with you to treat low blood glucose.

Diabetes medications that can cause low blood glucose are sulfonylureas, meglitinides, and insulin. While the meglitinides—nateglinide (Starlix) and repaglinide (Prandin)—lower blood glucose, the effect is not as dramatic as with the sul-

Table 4-1. Oral Diabetes Medications

Generic Name	Available as Generic?	Brand Name
alpha-Glucosidase Inhibitors		
acarbose	no	Precose
miglitol	no	Glyset
Biguanides		
metformin	yes	Glucophage
metformin (long-acting)	yes	Glucophage XR
metformin (liquid)	no	Riomet
Meglitinides		
nateglinide	no	Starlix
repaglinide	no	Prandin
Sulfonylureas		
acetohexamide	yes	generic only
chlorpropamide	yes	Diabinese
glimepiride	no	Amaryl
glipizide	yes	Glucotrol
glipizide (long-acting)	yes	Glucotrol XL
glyburide	yes	DiaBeta, Micronase
glyburide (micronized)	yes	Glynase PresTab
tolazamide	yes	generic only
tolbutamide	yes	generic only
Thiazolidinediones		
pioglitazone	no	Actos
rosiglitazone	no	Avandia
Combination Pills		
metformin + glyburide	yes	Glucovance
metformin + rosiglitazone	no	Avandamet
metformin + glipizide	no	Metaglip

Adapted from *The Diabetes Forecast Resource Guide*, 2006

Table 4-2. Action of Oral Diabetes Medication

Class	Site of Action	Action
Biguanides	Liver	Keep the liver from releasing too much glucose and also make muscle cells more sensitive to insulin.
Thiazolidinediones (TZDs)	Muscle cells	Make muscle cells more sensitive to insulin.
alpha-Glucosidase Inhibitors	Intestine	Slow the digestion of some carbohydrates. After-meal blood glucose peaks aren't as high.
Sulfonylureas	Pancreas	Stimulate pancreas to secrete more insulin.
Meglitinides	Pancreas	Stimulate pancreas to secrete more insulin, much like sulfonylureas, but are shorter in action.

Adapted from *The Diabetes Forecast Resource Guide*, 2006

fonylureas. However, they should still be taken with meals. If you have to skip the meal, skip the pill.

The sulfonylureas are:

- Glimepiride (Amaryl)
- Glipizide (Glucotrol) and glipizide long-acting (Glucotrol XL)
- Glyburide (DiaBeta, Micronase)
- Glyburide micronized (Glynase PresTab)
- Tolbutamide (generic)
- Tolazamide (generic)
- Chlorpropamide (Diabinese)
- Acetohexamide (generic)

The other diabetes pills do not cause low blood glucose when taken by themselves. But, when you take two different pills (or pills and insulin), your risk of having low blood glucose increases.

Be alert for feelings of shakiness, nervousness, irritability, and sweat. These are some of the warning signs that your blood glucose is dropping below normal. Your glucose could be low from taking too much diabetes medication, a skipped meal, extra exercise, a drug interaction between your diabetes medication and another medication you are taking, or a change in the way your kidneys or liver are working. Check your blood glucose and if you are experiencing low blood glucose, take 10–15 g of quickly absorbed carbohydrate, such as 1/2 cup of milk or orange juice, 2 teaspoonfuls of sugar, 5 or 6 Lifesavers, or 3 glucose tablets. Some diabetes pills slow down the absorption of carbohydrate, such as acarbose (Precose) and miglitol (Glyset). For these, you will need to use glucose products, milk, juice, or sugared sodas instead of solid food to bring your blood glucose back up. Glucose products come in tablet, gel, and liquid forms (see the box on page 51).

WHAT IF YOU FORGET TO TAKE A PILL?

For most oral diabetes medications, you can take a missed dose as soon as you remember it. If it is almost time to take the next dose, just take that dose on time—do not take a double dose. However, the case is different for some diabetes pills that should be taken with meals. If you miss a dose of repaglinide (Prandin) or nateglinide (Starlix) and you take it between meals, you could end up with low blood glucose. So, don't take it between meals. If you miss a dose of acarbose (Precose) or miglitol (Glyset), you should just take the next pill at the next meal, since its job is to slow the absorption of high-starch carbohydrate foods.

TIME ZONE CHANGES

If you take pills to control your diabetes and will be traveling to a time zone 3 hours or more from your own, you may have to change the time you take your medication. Discuss this with your health care provider and write down the instructions so you can take them with you. If you are told to take your pills with meals, ask whether you should take a pill even if you have to skip a meal.

PHYSICAL ACTIVITY

When you are on vacation, your activity level may increase quite a bit and you may have problems with low blood glucose.

You may need to eat an extra snack between meals containing carbohydrate and protein, such as cheese and crackers or half a meat sandwich. Check your blood glucose every 4 hours and be aware that exercise can keep lowering blood glucose into the next day.

Many people are tempted to adjust their oral medication dose while they travel like they would with insulin. However, except for repaglinide (Prandin), nateglinide (Starlix), acarbose (Precose), or miglitol (Glyset), making adjustments to your dose does not have an immediate effect on your blood glucose level. It is more difficult to adjust oral meds than it is to lower insulin by a few units. Some diabetes pills may be cut in half. However, this does not mean that you will get a correct half dose, and it may alter the way your body is able to absorb and use the medication. Check with your pharmacist about the pills you take before cutting them in half.

Most oral diabetes medications do come in a variety of dosages. Ask your health care provider about the smaller-dose pills, and whether you might take them on the days that you are very active. For example, your normal dose of medication is a 10-mg pill at breakfast and 10-mg pill at dinner. That same medication may come in a 2.5-mg pill or a 5-mg pill. Request a prescription for the 2.5-mg pill. Instead of taking one 10-mg pill before breakfast and one 10-mg pill before dinner, you would take four 2.5-mg pills before breakfast and four 2.5-mg pills before dinner. Then on the days you are active and your blood glucose levels are running low, you could adjust your dosage by taking only three 2.5-mg pills before breakfast and three before dinner. You'll need to check your blood glucose frequently to help you decide whether you need to adjust your medication and by how much.

THE EFFECTS OF ILLNESS

People who have type 2 diabetes do not usually produce ketones in their urine, but if you have type 2 diabetes and become ill—especially if you have vomiting and diarrhea so that you are dehydrated—check your urine for ketones. It's the sign of a serious condition developing. If you

have ketones in your urine, contact a
health care provider right away.

Ketone Testing

If your blood glucose is 250 mg/dl or higher
and it cannot be explained by what you have
just eaten, check for ketones in your urine.

Equipment:
- Ketone test strip
- Cup or clean container for sample
- A watch or other timing device

1. Dip a ketone test strip in a urine sample or
   pass it through the stream of urine.

2. Time the test according to the directions
   on the package.

3. The strip will change colors if ketones are
   present. Compare the test strip to the
   color chart on the package.

4. Record the results and have them available when you call your health care
   provider for guidance.

Chapter Five

TRAVEL BY AUTO, PLANE, OR BOAT

TRAVEL BY AUTO

When you travel by auto, you can be on your own schedule in the comfort of your own car or one you have rented. You don't need to be as concerned about the size and type of suitcases you pack as long as they fit in the car. The number and types of meals and snacks that you can enjoy at a restaurant or rest stop is limited only by your imagination. Although a person with diabetes can certainly travel alone, it is a good idea to have a traveling companion to share the driving, if possible.

It is important to be responsible for your diabetes while behind the wheel. Decide ahead of time how long you will drive before you stop to stretch—about every 2 hours is a good plan. Check your blood glucose before you start to drive—even if you have just eaten—and at each rest stop to be sure it doesn't drop too low while you are driving, which increases your risk of having an accident. Keep rapid-acting carbohydrate, such as fruit juice boxes or glucose tablets, on the seat next to you in case you need them.

Driving Tips for People with Diabetes

- To prevent fatigue, stop at regular intervals and stretch. Not only does this help your circulation, but it also protects you from the hypnosis-like effect caused by long drives.

- Take a cellular phone with you in the car for any emergencies that may arise. If you do not have a cell phone, you can buy one with prepaid minutes, like a calling card. The minutes can be renewed as needed. Even when not traveling, having a cell phone with you for emergencies is a good idea.

- Keep identification on you and in the car stating that you have diabetes. If you have an accident, you want everyone who comes to your aid to know that you have diabetes.

Contact AAA to get detailed maps of the area you will be visiting. Mapping websites can also provide detailed information and provide directions from one point to another. Be aware that while AAA or other auto clubs will provide you with information on construction, many websites that provide directions do not. Calling local police departments in areas you will be traveling will provide you with information on construction. Be sure to also pack a general map or atlas of the states you will be traveling through. Both you and your traveling companions should be familiar with the maps before you leave. A flashlight and extra batteries will help you read the maps or find items in the car during dusk and night driving without having to turn on the overhead light and disturb the driver.

Your feet and how they travel

When you sit in a car for several hours, your feet swell because fluids pool in them. That's why it's good to stop every few hours, walk around, and stretch; it helps your circulation and decreases the

On the Web

www.aaa.com

The website for AAA contains a lot of useful information for auto travelers, such as maps, road updates, safety tips, and even discounts and coupons. Be aware that some areas require AAA membership for access.

www.mapquest.com

This is one of the most popular mapping websites on the internet. Get detailed maps, driving directions, distance between destinations, approximate driving times, and destination information.

www.maps.google.com

This is the Google map site and it operates much like Mapquest.com, by providing detailed maps and directions. Unlike others, it also offers the ability to see satellite images of certain areas at different zoom levels.

swelling. If swelling becomes a problem, consider sitting in the rear seat when you are not driving and putting your feet up—higher than your heart if possible. Pack a few pillows to use to elevate your feet.

Even when you are sitting in the car and not walking, it is important to wear comfortable shoes and socks. Shoes with laces may be better because you can loosen them to allow for swelling. Never drive barefooted or in sandals.

Blood glucose levels

For many people, sitting in a car on a long trip will raise their blood glucose levels. High blood glucose can make you feel drowsy or irritable and may cause you to have blurred vision. If you already know that sitting in a car for long periods of time causes you to have high blood glucose, you may want to eat fewer carbohydrates at each meal. If you're driving, check your blood glucose at least every 2 hours.

If you take insulin and your blood glucose numbers are higher during your trip, you may want to increase your rapid-acting insulin (apidra, lispro, or novolog) by 1 or 2 units before meals. Discuss how to do this with your health care provider or diabetes educator. Choose one or the other—either limit your carbs at meals or increase your insulin, but don't do both at the same time or you'll risk going too low.

> ! ● If you get high blood glucose levels while driving for extended periods, either lower your carb intake or increase your insulin, but do not do both!

Most important of all, you must check for low blood glucose. If you have low blood glucose, you cannot respond quickly to what is happening on the road, and you are at increased risk for having an accident. Do not rely on how you feel. It is important to check your blood glucose at least every 2 hours to know exactly where it is. Be sure to always have snacks, such as juice or raisins and glucose tablets or gel (see the box *Over-the-Counter Products to Treat Low Blood Glucose* on page 51) to treat low blood glucose on the seat within your reach.

What if you get low while driving?

If you think you are having low blood glucose while you are driving, take 15–30 g of carbohydrate, such as one juice box or three glucose tablets, and immediately find a place to pull off the road. Check your blood glucose. Do not drive until all your symptoms are gone and your blood glucose has returned to normal (higher than 80 mg/dl). If it is time for a meal, take the time to eat. If you have a driving companion, this is the time to change drivers. Keep a cooler with you in the car with meals and snacks in it. Always pack a meal that can be eaten if you cannot find a restaurant, get into a traffic jam, or get lost. Pack twice as much food as you think you'll need. Try to keep your meals on schedule to prevent high blood glucose and low blood glucose.

Taking care of your insulin, Symlin, and Byetta

If you take insulin, Symlin, or Byetta, you need to keep it from getting too hot or too cold. These injectable medications can be kept in the food cooler as long as they're not touching ice, or you may keep them in a cool pack (see the box *Carrying Cases with an Insulin Cool Pack* on page 61). Keep all injectable medications with you inside the car, not in the trunk, where it can get too hot or cold. When you leave your car, take the medication with you, even if it is in the cooler. You may want to keep it in a little cooler of its own; on the very off chance that your car is stolen, you will still have your medication and blood glucose monitoring equipment.

Taking care of your eyes

Wearing sunglasses helps you avoid glare and protects your eyes. If you wear contacts, be sure to bring extra lenses and lens solution with you. It is also a good idea to bring prescription glasses and sunglasses in case you are unable to wear your contact lenses for any reason.

Car Travel Checklist

Keep these items with you in the car.

- ✓ Blood glucose monitoring supplies
- ✓ Insulin and supplies
- ✓ Insulin cool pack
- ✓ Cooler
- ✓ Snacks
- ✓ Meal in cooler
- ✓ Glucose tablets or other quick-acting glucose
- ✓ Bottles of water
- ✓ Other fluids, such as sugar-free soda and juice

- ✓ Sunglasses
- ✓ Cellular phone
- ✓ Maps
- ✓ Flashlight and batteries
- ✓ Medic alert ID in car and on person
- ✓ Comfortable shoes and socks
- ✓ Pillow
- ✓ Blanket
- ✓ Sweater or light jacket

In the trunk

Any items that are kept in the trunk should be things that you can wait to get to at regularly scheduled stops. You can pack bottled water or a container of water that you can refill at rest stops. Freeze the bottles before you leave on the trip. This will keep the water cold during much of the trip. It can also keep other items in a cooler cold. You can also pack other types of fluids in your cooler, such as sugar-free drinks or juice.

TRAVEL BY PLANE

Traveling by airplane is usually the quickest way to get to your destination. Most flights are on time, but you should be prepared for delayed or cancelled flights and lost baggage. Carry all your diabetes supplies and important papers. The contents of your carry-on bag (see chapter 2) will help make your trip go smoothly. Even if security situations restrict certain items, you should always be able to get your insulin, oral medication, or other diabetes supplies with you on the plane. Also bring all the food that you might need with you. Airlines rarely provide meals any more. You may have the opportunity to purchase a snack if the flight is over 90 minutes, but the snacks may not meet your dietary needs. It is best to pack your own meal. If you are flying first class and the travel time is over 90 minutes, a meal may be served. You can ask the travel agent or airline when you make your reservation.

When booking your flights, try to get a direct flight. If you must take a flight with a connection, look at the in-flight airline magazine for the map of the airport where you have to change planes. This can help you find the gate for your next flight more quickly. If the distance is manageable, the walk will

On the Web

www.<AirlineName>.com

Obviously, this isn't a website. But if you replace <AirlineName> with the name of the airline on which you're traveling, you'll more than likely get that airline's website. For instance, *www.nwa.com* is the website for Northwest Airlines, while typing *www.americanairlines.com* will take you to the website of American Airlines.

provide you with some exercise after sitting for a long time.

If you are concerned that the distance between the two gates or to the baggage claim is greater than you are able to walk, request wheelchair or motor cart assistance. You can do this ahead of time over the phone or when you check in. You can also request assistance at the gate before departure for when you land. A notation will be put in the computer so that some one meets you at your destination. The flight attendant can also request a wheelchair or motor cart to get you to your gate prior to the plane landing. An airline representative will meet you and take you to your connecting gate. The airline is happy to help you with this, so don't let embarrassment keep you from taking good care of yourself.

Where do you want to sit?

Request a bulkhead or emergency exit aisle seat. These seats have maximum legroom, and it will be easier for you to get up and move around periodically. Be aware that if you choose an exit row seat, there are responsibilities to help other passengers in case of an emergency. If you have any disabilities that would not allow you to assist other passengers, the exit row is not an option for you. An aisle seat on any row would be the next best choice. On longer flights, take the opportunity to get out of your seat and stretch. When the aisles are clear, walk up and down to keep your circulation moving and decrease swelling in your feet. Be sure to wear comfortable shoes that allow you to wear socks. Often flights are cool and socks will keep your feet warm. You can always

A Little More Leg Room

As of the printing of this edition, some airlines are offering options for extra leg room. NWA will seat you in select seats in the aisle and exit row close to the front of the plane for an extra $15 at check-in. For $299 per year, United Airlines offers a program that guarantees you and a traveling companion on the same itinerary an aisle seat toward the front of the plane. Other airlines are offering similar deals, so check around and see what's being offered. Call your airline or check their website for more information.

carry another pair of shoes to change into at your destination if you are going to a warm climate.

When you board the airplane, take a blanket from the overhead compartments. There are not enough for all passengers, so it's first come first served. You might want to cover your legs and feet with the blanket. Many airlines no longer have pillows. So purchasing a travel pillow may be helpful. On long flights, folding the blanket and using it to elevate your legs will help with circulation and decrease swelling in your feet.

Dry as a desert

The air inside the airplane is dry. Carry an empty sports water bottle. with you on the plane The flight attendant can fill it for you from the bottled water in the galley or from the beverage cart. Drink plenty of non-sweetened fluids. Avoid alcohol and limit caffeine. This will help prevent dehydration. If allowed on the plane, carry lip balm and hand cream and apply them during the flight.

Onboard diabetes care

Carry food and snacks with you to get you through the flight and prevent low blood glucose. Remember that when you are inactive, your blood glucose may be higher than usual. It is important to check your blood glucose on a regular basis while you're flying.

Many airplane restrooms have a section of the wall designed for you to dispose of your insulin syringes and lancets safely. You may also choose to put your used equipment back in your carry-on bag to be disposed of when you reach your destination. Do not dispose of them in the regular trash or on your meal tray.

What if you cannot travel?

Each airline has their own policy regarding flight changes or cancellations if you become ill prior to traveling or while you are traveling. Be sure to ask the airline or your travel agent for the policy of the airline you will be using. Get the policy in writing. Also get the names of contact people and phone numbers at the airlines that are available 24 hours a day in case

Frequent Flyer Perks

If you are a frequent flyer or have access to points or coupons to upgrade to first class, this will be helpful on longer flights. First-class seats are larger and provide more legroom. Often the seat works like a recliner chair and the leg rest can elevate your feet. Meal service is more frequent and more predictable because there are fewer passengers to serve and the food is of a higher quality.

you need assistance in changing your flights because you are ill. You can also ask your travel agent about getting trip insurance, which will reimburse you for trips or tours that you had to cancel and the airlines or the tour company would not cover.

A helping hand

If you will be bringing your own wheelchair, walker, or cane, the airlines will make arrangements to help you to your seat and store your equipment. When your flight lands, your equipment will be returned to you and you will be assisted off the flight. Let the airlines know when you make your flight arrangements of any special needs you have. When you check in, tell them again that you will need special assistance. You will find that you are given first-class treatment in these situations, so don't be hesitant about asking.

Air sick?

After a discussion with your health care provider, take medication such as Dramamine (pills) or Scopolamine (patches) with you to prevent motion sickness. It is best to take (or apply) them 30 minutes before you fly. These medications will usually make you drowsy.

More about luggage

Most luggage arrives at your destination without delay; however, if your bag does not appear on the carousel after all the luggage has been unloaded, go to the airline office located in the baggage claim area and report your missing luggage. The airline will want to know exactly what your bag looked like, what you have in it, and how it was labeled. Always put an identification tag on your luggage. It is also a good idea to label the inside of your luggage, too, just in case your luggage tag comes off. Most delays are caused because your luggage did not get on your flight either at the beginning or on the switch to a connecting flight. Usually your luggage will arrive on the next scheduled flight. While this may cause you some inconvenience, if you have packed your carry-on bag carefully, you will have enough supplies to get you through until your luggage arrives.

When your luggage arrives at the airport, the airline will deliver it to you. If

On the Web

www.luggagefree.com

If you don't feel like lugging all your bags with you, or you're worried about the airline losing your bags, then this website may be just what you're looking for. Luggage-Free is a luggage delivery service that ships your luggage directly from your home to your destination.

Prices run from $2 per pound for air delivery (2 business days) to $1 per pound for ground (4–5 business days), plus pick-up fee. International services are also available. Visit the website or call 1-800-361-6871 for more information.

your luggage is lost and not recovered, you can make a claim to the airlines to replace what you have lost. On domestic flights, federal regulations limit the amount an airline must pay you to $250 for your lost or damaged luggage and its contents. If the contents of your luggage are worth more, then you may declare this at check-in, up to the airlines maximum coverage, which usually is between $250 and $500. The airline will ask you to pay an additional fee to obtain this extra coverage. You might consider flight insurance or trip insurance to cover your luggage, depending on the value of its contents. Be sure to pack jewelry and other valuable items in your carry-on baggage.

On international flights, coverage for missing or damaged luggage is covered by the Warsaw Convention. Damages are calculated based on the weight of your luggage. The value of your lost luggage is reimbursed at the rate of $9.07 per pound. If your luggage was not weighed prior to departing, then the airline will assume that all of your luggage weighed 70 pounds, and you will be reimbursed

$634.90. There are time limits for when you may make a claim, so check your luggage for missing or damaged goods, and report it immediately to the airline.

Airplane Travel Checklist

For your carry-on bag:

✓ Airline tickets

✓ Passport

✓ Hotel reservation information

✓ Car rental information

✓ Other important papers

✓ Jewelry or other valuables

✓ Blood glucose monitoring supplies

✓ Insulin and supplies

✓ Insulin cool pack

✓ All medications

✓ Snacks

✓ Glucose tablets or other quick-acting glucose

✓ Map of airport you are connecting through

✓ Medic Alert in your tote and one on your person

✓ Comfortable shoes and socks

✓ Sweater or lightweight jacket

✓ Dramamine (pills) or Scopolamine (patches) for air sickness

TRAVEL BY BOAT

Cruises

Most cruises usually combine airline travel with sea travel in order for you to get to your port of departure. When you choose your cruise, you will have the opportunity to pick your cabin. You will need to decide what type of bed you want and on which deck you want your cabin. Most cruise lines have pictures with descriptions and diagrams of the ship. Ask to see the diagram to help you make your decision. If you have a tendency for seasickness, you might prefer a cabin that is well above the water level. If you have trouble walking or have any handicap that will make it difficult to get around, you should choose a cabin near the dining rooms. Work with your travel agent or the cruise line to pick the cabin that will best suit your special needs.

Menus for meals are prepared before departure. Most cruise lines offer many choices at each meal, and there are opportunities to eat more than three meals per day. Passengers are assigned a seating time for dinner, but other meals usually have a range of times you can eat. Your travel agent or the cruise line can provide you with a list of meal times and menus that you can review before traveling. If your diabetes program requires you to eat at a specific time each day, be sure to request the meal times when you choose your cruise and request a specific seating for dinner. Although the meals on a cruise offer you a great deal of variety, you may request special meals at this time as well.

Check ahead of time to see if your cabin will have a small refrigerator to store your insulin and other injectable medications. If you do not have a refrigerator in your cabin, your extra insulin can be stored in the refrigerator of the medical clinic on the ship. Keep the insulin you are using in an insulin cool pack (see the box on page 61). The cool pack inserts can be frozen in the refrigerator of the medical facility.

What if you become ill?

Ask specifically about the cruise line's cancellation policy or reimbursement policy if you are ill prior to the trip and are unable to travel. Also, ask about their policy if you become ill during the trip and must leave the trip early. Obtain the policy in writing. Ask for phone numbers and names of individuals you can contact directly. Most cruise line policies are fairly rigid. You want to be sure you understand the policies of the cruise line before you put down a deposit.

Determine what arrangements can be made to fly you home from one of the ports of call if you are ill. You may need to purchase special trip insurance to protect yourself. You may also wish to obtain a credit card that covers illness and special or medical care of the owner while traveling. For example, the Platinum American Express card or a Gold MasterCard generally covers these costs and the costs of having you airlifted home. Call your credit card company to see what travel benefits you may have.

Settling in

When you have settled into your cabin, introduce yourself to the health care team in the ship's medical facility. Most ships have a physician and nursing staff on board for the duration of the trip. They can be helpful if you become ill on the trip.

Be sure to keep snacks or a form of glucose in your cabin to treat low blood glucoses or if you need food before you go to sleep. Food is readily available during the day for mid-morning or afternoon snacks if needed. Always carry a form of glucose with you in case you need to treat low blood glucose (see the box on page 51). The ship is big, so do not count on being able to get back to your room to treat low blood glucose.

Let's get physical

Pack comfortable clothes and shoes. There will be plenty of opportunities to get exercise on the ship. In addition to using the indoor health club, you may walk around the decks. Most ships also have swimming pools you can use.

In the sun

Remember that the sun can be stronger when it reflects off the water. Use sunscreen, sunglasses, and a sun hat. You might want to wear lightweight long-sleeve clothing for part of the day to protect yourself from overexposure to the sun. Be aware that sunbathing may cause low blood glucose.

Motion sickness?

Be sure to carry medication for motion sickness. You may wish to take this if the cruise is rough or at the first sign of motion sickness. If the pills or the patch does not work and you are vomiting, then try a suppository such as Tigan, which should be in your first aid kit (page 35). If the vomiting persists longer than an hour after you have inserted the suppository, go to the medical facility. The health care providers will be able to give you an injection of Tigan or another medication to stop the vomiting. Depending on how long you have been vomiting, you might also need fluid replacement through an intravenous line. This can be done at the medical facility.

When you go to see the sights

Many cruise ships stop at different ports for passengers to go sightseeing. Pack a bag of necessities when you go. Be sure to take your blood glucose meter, insulin or diabetes pills, and any other medications you will need while you are gone. Take a snack (such as cheese and crackers or half a sandwich) with you and glucose to treat low blood glucose. And pack at least one bottle of water. Put on sunscreen before you leave and take the bottle with you. Take your sunglasses and a sun hat. Be sure to wear good walking shoes. Carry your letter that says you have diabetes and need to carry your blood glucose meter, lancets, and, if needed, syringes. You should always wear a medic alert ID.

The cruise director should be able to tell you about places to eat safely while you are sightseeing. Leave enough time to get back to the ship, so you are not left at port!

Cruise Ship Checklist

Keep these things with you on board ship and at ports of call:

✓ Blood glucose monitoring supplies

✓ Insulin and other injectable medications for the day

✓ Cool pack

✓ Other medications as needed

✓ Glucose tablet or other quick-acting glucose

✓ Sunscreen

✓ Sunglasses

✓ Sun hat

✓ Comfortable shoes and socks

✓ Medic alert ID on person and supplies

✓ Dramamine (pills) or Scopolamine (patches) for motion sickness

✓ Snacks

✓ Bottle of water

✓ Letter indicating that you have diabetes and need to carry blood glucose supplies, insulin, and other supplies with you at all times

Chapter Six

EATING WELL & EXERCISING ON THE ROAD

Eating well while traveling and being away from home can be challenging. You'll need to give some thought to time changes, availability of food, variety of food, how food is prepared, and portion sizes. Unless you have a kitchen and you can prepare some of your meals, you will be eating out for all three meals, so it's time to sharpen your eating-out skills. This chapter has suggestions to help you choose wisely from a variety of cuisines. To balance the blood glucose effect of the delicious (we hope) meals that you will be having, travel also offers an abundance of opportunities to get much more exercise than you usually do.

TIME CHANGES

It is best to get yourself accustomed to the time zone you are visiting as quickly as possible. If you go to bed, get up, and eat your meals based on the time where you are, you will adjust more quickly. Of course, it may not always be quite that simple. In some countries, it is customary to eat meals at a later time. Or the big meal of the day is the noon meal rather than the evening meal. You can make adjustments for this. If you take insulin or oral medication specifically for the dinner meal, but you will be eating your larger meal at the noon hour, consider taking your rapid-acting insulin before the noon meal instead. If you are on an insulin pump, simply switch the dinner insulin bolus with the lunchtime insulin bolus. The same would be true of the oral medication designed to cover just your dinner meal. See Table 6-1 for more about making adjustments to your medication for time changes, and discuss them with your health care practitioners.

Table 6-1. Adjusting Diabetes Medications for Mealtime Changes

Present Program (Largest meal dinner)	Changes (Largest meal lunch)
Insulin	
Two injections daily	
20 units NPH at breakfast 10 units Humalog, Novolog, or Apidra at breakfast	No change
20 units NPH at dinner	10 units Humalog, Novolog, or Apidra at lunch
10 units Humalog, Novolog, or Apidra at dinner	20 units NPH at dinner
Three injections daily	
20 units NPH, Lantus, or Levimir at breakfast 10 units Humalog, Novolog, or Apdria at breakfast	No change
10 units Humalog, Novolog, or Apidra at dinner	10 units Humalog, Novolog, or Apidra at lunch
20 units NPH, Lantus, or Levimir at bedtime	No change

(cont. on next page)

Present Program (Largest meal dinner)	Changes (Largest meal lunch)
Four injections daily	
20 units NPH, Lantus, or Levimir 10 units Humalog, Novolog, or Apidra at breakfast	No change
10 units Humalog, Novolog, or Apidra at lunch	Take at dinner
14 units Humalog, Novolog, or Apidra at dinner	Take at lunch
20 units NPH, Lantus, or Levimir at bedtime	No change
Four injections daily (basal/bolus)	
10 units Humalog, Novolog, or Apidra at breakfast	No change
10 units Humalog, Novolog, or Apidra at lunch	Take at dinner
14 units Humalog, Novolog, or Apidra at dinner	Take at lunch
20 units Lantus or Levimir at bedtime	No change

Insulin Pump Therapy

Switch bolus taken at dinner with bolus taken at lunch.

Oral Diabetes Medication

Continue to take as prescribed.

If your dinner will be served several hours later than you usually eat, you may need to have a snack at the time you would ordinarily have dinner. Then, since dinner will be later, you may be able to skip a bedtime snack. But don't guess; check your blood glucose before bed to see if you need a snack.

HOW WILL YOU EAT WHILE YOU'RE AWAY?

Where will you eat?

When you arrive at your destination, check out the availability of grocery stores, markets, and restaurants or other places to eat. Find out how far you will need to travel to get to these places and what transportation you can use to get there. Also ask about the hours of operation. For example, over the Easter weekend in European countries, all the grocery stores are closed for several days.

When you go out to eat, carry your blood glucose meter and insulin or diabetes pills with you. Do not take your insulin, Symlin, Byetta, or other medications until you are sure when your food will be served. You might want to wait until the food is actually on the table before taking your medication.

What will you eat?

Most restaurants offer a wide variety of foods. You can usually get the carbohydrates you need from breads, pasta, rice, potatoes, and fruit. Do not hesitate to ask questions about how dishes are prepared or about serving sizes. This is part of the service that you are paying for. Ask how foods are prepared. Ask about low-fat or fat-free salad dressings. (Be aware that fat-free salad dressings may have more carbohydrate than the regular dressing, so they will have an effect on your blood glucose, especially if you have several servings.)

You may request to have your foods prepared in a way different from what is listed on the menu. Fried foods can be broiled. Sauces and gravies can be served on the side. You will want to know if a sauce has sugar in it or is high in fat, because these ingredients will affect your blood glucose. Ask questions and you will help your waiter or waitress learn a little about diabetes, too.

As more and more people eat out at restaurants, restaurant owners have become more health-conscious, and most menus have "lite" or "healthy" entrees. Most eating places offer sugar substitutes, diet beverages, fruit juice, and decaffeinated coffee and tea. Some have reduced-calorie salad dressings, low-fat or fat-free milk, and salt substitutes. But even if they don't offer special meals, it is pretty easy to find salads, fish and seafood, vegetables, baked or broiled food, and whole-grain breads. See Table 6-2 for more suggestions on healthy food choices.

How much will you eat?

More often than not, restaurants serve very large portions. This is generally too much food for one person. You may be able to order a half portion or share your entree with a friend or family member. Before you begin to eat, decide how much of the food on your plate meets your real needs. Do not be afraid to leave food on your plate.

Table 6-2. Healthy Choices for Eating Out

Green Light	Red Light
Appetizers	
Clear broth, bouillon	Cream soups, thick soups
Fresh fruit, unsweetened	Canned fruit cocktail
Fresh steamed seafood	Breaded or fried seafood
Eggs	
Poached or boiled	Fried or scrambled
Salads	
Tossed vegetable	Coleslaw
Asparagus salad	Canned fruit, gelatin salads
Breads	
Whole-grain rolls, crackers	Sweet rolls, coffee cake
Biscuits, breads	Croissants
Potatoes, pasta, and rice	
Baked, boiled, or steamed potatoes	Fried, creamed, scalloped, or au gratin potatoes

Green Light	Red Light
Fats	
Low-calorie salad dressing	Regular salad dressing
Low-fat sour cream or yogurt	Regular sour cream, gravy, cream sauces
Vegetables	
Raw, stewed, steamed, or boiled	Creamed, scallloped, or au gratin
Meat, poultry, and fish	
Roasted, baked, broiled lean meats, skin or fat removed	Fried, battered, or breaded; cured meats; organ meats; stews and casseroles
Desserts	
Fresh fruit	Sweetened fruit, pudding, custard, pastries
Nonfat or low-fat frozen yogurt	Ice cream
Beverages	
Water, coffee, tea, fat-free milk, diet soda	Chocolate milk, cocoa, milkshakes, regular soft drinks

More restaurants are now offering menus that list calories and nutrients, or they'll provide this information if you request it. If you ask, chefs can sometimes create low-fat entrees just for you. Some cooks will remove the skin from a chicken, omit extra butter on the dish, broil instead of fry, and serve sauces on the side. There are restaurants that will allow you to order small portions at reduced prices, or you can share with someone else at the table. All these improvements make it easier to fit restaurant foods into your meal plan.

FOLLOWING THE PLAN

You want to feel healthy and energized on your trip, so it's a good idea to try to follow your meal plan as much as possible. Here are some tips to help you:

- If you can, pick a restaurant that offers a wide variety of choices.

- If you don't know the ingredients in a dish or the serving size, ask.

- Try to eat the same size servings that you eat at home.

- Ask that fish or meat be broiled with little added fat.

- Ask to have sour cream or butter for a baked potato on the side or not brought at all.

- If you are on a low-sodium diet or want to cut back, ask that no or little salt be added to your food.

- Ask to have sauces, gravy, and dressings served on the side.

- Avoid breaded or fried foods. If the food arrives breaded, you can peel off the outer coating or send it back if you ordered it without breading.

- Use the menu creatively. For instance, order the fruit cup appetizer or the breakfast melon for your dessert after dinner.

- Ask for substitutions, such as low-fat cottage cheese, baked potato instead of French fries, or a double portion of a vegetable instead of the fries.

- Ask about low-calorie items, such as salad dressings, even if they are not listed on the menu.

• Remember, you are the customer; it is okay to ask for what you need.

What about fast foods?

Today fast food restaurants are offering healthier choices, such as salads, baked potatoes, chili, and grilled chicken, which makes it easier to fit fast food into a healthy eating plan. But there are still plenty of high-fat, high-calorie fast food choices, so take care with what you order. It is possible to eat an entire day's worth of fat, salt, and calories in just one fast food meal.

Healthy Points to Consider

Follow the guidelines your dietitian or health care provider has given you. For instance, you may be counting calories, grams of carbs, or grams of fat. If you have not been given guidelines, try to keep these points in mind:

1. Eat a variety of foods in medium-sized amounts.

2. Eat more vegetables.

3. Limit your fat intake.

4. Watch the amount of sodium in the food choices.

Many fast food restaurants can give you the nutritional information of their foods if you ask. You can also visit their websites or consult a book of restaurant nutrition facts. By knowing the nutritional value of the fast food, you can choose ones that will fit into your meal plan. If you have some higher-fat fast food for one meal, try to eat low-fat foods like fruits and vegetables for your other meals that day. Balance is important. Here are some tips to help you choose among fast foods:

☞ For breakfast, try a plain bagel, toast, or English muffin. Drink fruit juice or low-fat milk. Order cold cereal with skim milk, pancakes without butter, or plain scrambled eggs. Limit or pass up the bacon and sausage.

☞ Load up on lettuce and vegetables at a salad bar. Go easy on the dressing, bacon bits, cheeses, croutons, mayonnaise, and macaroni salads. Too much of even a low-calorie salad dressing can make a difference. Check the number of calories on the packet.

☞ Order regular (or junior-size) sandwiches rather than the jumbo, giant, or deluxe sandwiches to get fewer calories and less fat, cholesterol, and sodium.

☞ Choose lean roast beef, lean ham, or turkey or chicken breast sandwiches.

☞ Skip the buttery croissant and eat your sandwich on a bun or bread instead to save calories and fat.

☞ Choose chicken or fish if it is roasted, unbreaded, grilled, baked, or broiled without fat. Chicken or fish that is battered, breaded, or fried is higher in calories and fat than a hamburger.

☞ Stay away from double burgers or super hot dogs with cheese, chili, or sauces. Cheese can carry an extra 100 calories, as well as extra fat and sodium.

☞ Order items without toppings, rich sauces, or mayonnaise. Add lettuce, tomato, onion, and mustard instead.

☞ Choose cheese pizza with vegetables. Toppings such as pepperoni, sausage, and extra cheese add calories, fat, and sodium. A word of caution: the high carbohydrate content of pizza can make blood glucose levels go really high in some people, but the high fat content of pizza may delay the blood glucose rise until several hours later. Check your blood glucose at different times after eating pizza to learn how it affects you.

☞ Order tacos, tostados, bean burritos, soft tacos, and other non-fried items in Mexican restaurants. Choose chicken over beef. Avoid beans refried in lard. Pile on extra lettuce, tomatoes, and salsa. Go easy on cheese, sour cream, and guacamole. Watch out for the deep-fried taco salad shell; a taco salad can have more than 1,000 calories!

☞ If you have room for dessert, go for sugar-free nonfat frozen yogurt. Ices, sorbets, and sherbets do have less fat and fewer calories than ice cream, but they are full of sugar and can raise your blood glucose too high unless you work the extra sugar into your meal plan. Some fast food places now offer fresh fruit!

☞ Sugar-free cookies, cakes, candies, and ice cream often have the same or more calories than regular foods do. The sweeteners used may also elevate your blood glucose in the same way as regular foods. If you wish to have cookies, cakes, candies, or ice cream, consider using the regular foods but limit the portion size and the frequency that you eat them.

☞ Remember that fat-free foods do not mean calorie free. If you choose to include an item that is fat free, be sure to read the label so you know what the total calories and carbohydrates are in a portion.

☞ When reading a label, it is important to look at the calories, fat, and carbohydrate per portion. Then look at how many portions per container. This is the tricky part. For instance, a small container of cookies may be 100 calories per portion, but the portion size is two cookies. And there are six cookies per container. If you ate all six cookies you would be eating 300 calories.

By making the right choices and balancing the meals when you eat out, you can enjoy yourself and take care of your diabetes at the same time.

PHYSICAL ACTIVITY

If you've done quite a bit of walking or physical activity during the day, be aware that it will continue to lower your blood glucose for hours afterward. This is one of the glorious benefits of exercise. When you walk all day or do a lot of physical activity, you will need an extra snack between meals containing protein and carbohydrate, such as cheese and crackers or half a meat sandwich. If you are very active, you may want to decrease your diabetes medication

---

On the Web

www.nutritiondata.com

There are many online restaurant nutrition fact counters out there and they're all worth checking out. But this website also offers additional nutrition analysis of specific foods, showing how healthy certain items are and ranking them by how well they fit into healthy eating plans. For the most up-to-date nutrition information from specific restaurants, visit that restaurant's site.

to prevent low blood glucose. Use your glucose monitor to help you decide. And discuss this possibility with your health care provider before you go.

Exercise and insulin

If you are on insulin, eat a protein and carbohydrate snack as needed during the day, and first try lowering your insulin doses by 10%. Check your blood glucose levels the first day of activity, and decide whether you need to lower your insulin the next day by an additional 10%. Be aware that the glucose-lowering effects of exercise may carry over into the night or the next day. Since you can't be sure how much your blood glucose levels will drop from increasing your activity level, go ahead and check your blood glucose more often. Always carry quick-acting carbohydrates, such as fruit juice or glucose tablets, with you to treat low blood glucose if it occurs. You may need a bedtime snack. It's healthier to lower your insulin dose than to have to worry about unexpected low blood glucose and then have to eat to raise your blood glucose level.

Exercise and diabetes pills

If you are taking diabetes pills that can cause low blood glucose, you need to be aware of the effect that increased physical activity has on your blood glucose level. If you check your blood glucose and find it is low, eat a snack containing protein and carbohydrate. If you'll be hiking all day, for example, you may need to eat several snacks over the day.

Some wonder whether they can simply lower their dose of medication. However, except for repaglinide (Prandin), acarbose (Precose), miglitol (Glyset), or nateglinide (Starlix), making adjustments to your oral meds does not have an immediate effect on your blood glucose level. See the section on adjusting oral medications in chapter 4 for more on this.

ENJOY

The three Es of travel could well be eating, exercise, and enjoyment. With a little planning ahead, you can easily have all three. And create many pleasant memories of your trip.

Chapter Seven

ILLNESS DURING YOUR TRIP

Taking the right precautions to prevent illness is the best way to stay healthy and enjoy your trip. However, if you do get sick, you need to be able to respond quickly and know when and where to seek help. You can pack medications to treat common illnesses, such as colds or diarrhea (page 35). If you haven't already, talk with your provider about making a plan for sick-day care (see the box *Sick-Day Care*), and be sure to take it with you. When you arrive at your destination, find out where the nearest health care center and pharmacy are located. Contact the ADA at 1-800-DIABETES

(1-800-342-2383) or *www.diabetes.org* if
you need help locating health care in the
United States.

If you are traveling in a foreign country,
call the U.S. Consulate or U.S. Embassy
when you arrive or visit *www.istm.org* for
unofficial information. If you will be in
the area for an extended period of time,
give the consulate your phone number
and tell them how you can be reached.
The primary job of the consular officer is
to help U.S. citizens traveling abroad, so
they can help you in many ways, especially
if you become ill and need assistance.
They have lists of doctors and health care
facilities in the area.

WHAT CAN YOU DO BEFORE YOU GO?

Before you travel to foreign countries, it's
a good idea to schedule a travel medical
interview at a travel health clinic. The
interview and visit will address your trav-
el-related needs. Based on where you will
be traveling, the health care providers will
advise you of health risks, the types of
medications you should take with you,

Sick-Day Care

What to do if you are too sick to eat:

1. Measure your blood glucose every 2 hours and record the result.

2. Call your health care provider for assistance. If you are unable to reach him or her, take at least half your dose of insulin.

3. Drink fluids every 2 hours. Select fluids from the choices listed below and sip them slowly over a 2-hour period. Use ice chips; you may tolerate this fluid better.

   - 1 cup (8 oz) regular soda (not diet soda)

   - 1 cup (8 oz) fruit juice

   - 2 cups (16 oz) Gatorade

   - Sweetened tea (2 tsp sugar in 1 cup tea)

   AND

   - In addition to the above items, 1 cup of bouillon or (dried) chicken soup, with water

4. Drink additional water during the day or use ice chips to avoid dehydration.

5. Seek health care when:

   - Your blood glucose is 240 mg/dl or more and does not drop below 200 mg/dl when you use additional insulin

(cont. on next page)

- Your blood glucose is 240 mg/dl or more and there are ketones in your urine

- You feel too sick to eat, are unable to keep down food or fluids, and you feel you need help or advice

If you take diabetes pills, do not stop taking them. Ask your provider whether you should adjust the dosage for sick days. In general:

- Check your blood glucose levels more often—every 2 hours;

- Check for ketones if your blood glucose is 240 mg/dl or more;

- Use the food choices on page 162.

and any immunizations you need before you travel. Have this check-up several months before your trip. This will allow enough time for the travel clinic to review your medical history, order any needed tests, and give you any immunizations that you might need.

Immunizations

Not all health care providers have access to immunizations. Call ahead of time to see if your health care provider gives immunizations. You may need to go to the public health department or a special clinic for travel. Most immunizations are given in a series over several months. Be sure to allow enough time to get the whole series. Before the visit, check your records to determine which immunizations you have had and when you got them. Also, know the date of your last tetanus shot. They are good for 10 years in adults, and this is a good time to update your tetanus if you need to.

Keep a record of all of your immunizations. The health clinic or your health care provider can provide you with a small booklet for recording the types of immunizations you have had and the dates you got them. Keep this record of your immunizations with your other important documents while traveling.

Be sure to have a flu shot each year. People with diabetes are four times more likely to die of complications of the flu or pneumonia than people who do not have diabetes. The vaccine may not prevent you from getting the flu, but it will minimize your symptoms and the length of your ill-

ness if you do get it. You should also get a
pneumonia vaccine. After the initial vaccine, you should have a booster shot every
5–6 years.

DO YOU NEED TO CHECK YOUR BLOOD GLUCOSE WHEN YOU ARE SICK?

Yes. In fact, if you are ill, you need to
check your blood glucose more frequently
than usual. If you take insulin, you may
need to increase your insulin to keep your
blood glucose in the normal range. If your
blood glucose is low because you are
unable to eat, you may need to lower your
insulin dose. Do not stop taking your
insulin when you are ill. It is best to work
out a sick-day plan with your provider or
educator before you travel that will include
how to make adjustments to your insulin
(see the box *Sick-Day Insulin Adjustments*).

Insulin Supplements for Sick Days

When you are sick, your blood glucose
levels will begin to rise and you may need
more insulin. To compensate for this

problem, you will need to add extra rapid-acting insulin to your usual doses of insulin until your blood glucose levels return to normal. The guidelines below are suggested adjustments; work with your health care provider to determine how you should adjust your insulin for sick days.

The dose of extra insulin is based on your blood glucose levels, so you must use your blood glucose meter. If you have ketones in your urine or blood, you'll need to double the dose of insulin listed below. Take the extra insulin before each meal, or if you are not eating meals, take it every 4 hours. Do not take extra insulin before bed because it could cause low blood glucose problems while you are asleep.

Be sure to measure your blood glucose every 2 hours. If your blood glucose is higher than 240 mg/dl, check your urine or blood for ketones. Keep a record of your blood glucose levels, ketone levels, your usual dose of insulin, and any extra insulin you take. Record the time, too.

Sick-Day Insulin Adjustments

For blood glucose of (mg/dl)	Add to normal insulin dose
Less than 200	0 units of Humalog, Novolog, or Apidra
200–249	2 units of Humalog, Novolog, or Apidra
250–299	3 units of Humalog, Novolog, or Apidra
300–349	4 units of Humalog, Novolog, or Apidra
350–399	5 units of Humalog, Novolog, or Apidra
400 or more	6 units of Humalog, Novolog, or Apidra

Double the extra dose of insulin if you have ketones present.

Adapted from "Sick Days," page 75, *Diabetes 101*, Brackenridge, et al.

WHAT DO YOU DO IF YOU ARE VOMITING?

If you are ill and vomiting, you must be sure that you do not get dehydrated. You will need to take in fluids to prevent this from happening. You have to strike a careful balance because drinking fluids may cause more vomiting, but you must not let yourself get dehydrated. If you are vomiting, you will need to adjust your meal plan. Although you need carbohydrates to prevent low blood glucose, solid food will just aggravate the problem. You need fluids that contain carbohydrate.

You can try converting your meal plan into liquids. Check your blood glucose every 2 hours. If your blood glucose is greater than 240 mg/dl, sip fluids that are sugar free, and check for ketones. If your blood glucose is less than 240 mg/dl, then drink fluids with 15 g of carbohydrate in them (see Table 7-1. *Fluids and Foods for when You Are Ill*).

You may control vomiting with a rectal suppository, such as Tigan. This is a prescription item and should be part of your first aid kit (see page 35). After you insert the Tigan, it usually begins to work in 30 minutes. Do not resume your normal meal plan yet. Continue to monitor your blood glucose every 2 hours and sip fluids. Most flu bugs will last 24–48 hours.

Table 7-1. Fluids and Foods for when You Are Ill

Contact a health care facility if you are having trouble eating or keeping foods down, and take your insulin. These easy-to-digest foods may be helpful when you are ill. Since you still take insulin, you should eat some carbohydrate every 2 hours throughout the day and night. The foods listed below each contain 15 g of carbohydrate.

Apple juice	1/2 cup
Grape juice	1/3 cup
Orange juice	1/2 cup
Gatorade	1 1/2 cup
Applesauce	1/2 cup
Cooked cereal	1/2 cup
Baked custard	1/2 cup
Saltines	6
Fruited yogurt	1/2 cup
Ice cream	1/2 cup
Pineapple juice	1/2 cup
Popsicle	1/2
Jello	1/3 cup
Thick soup	1/2 cup
Thin soup	1 cup
Regular soda	1/2 cup
Honey	3 tsp
Lifesavers	7
Milk	1 cup

You'll need extra calorie-free fluids to prevent dehydration. Use free liquids such as broth or water.

Be sure the flu is over before you begin eating solid food again.

If, despite all of your efforts, you are unable to control the vomiting, you may become dehydrated. Then it may be necessary for you to go to a medical clinic or hospital to get fluids intravenously. If you are vomiting without relief for 6 hours, seek medical care. If you are vomiting and not eating meals, you may need to take small amounts of insulin but avoid taking other medications, such as Symlin. Be sure to discuss this with your health care team.

WHAT DO YOU DO IF YOU HAVE VOMITING AND DIARRHEA?

If you have the flu and are vomiting and also have diarrhea, you will not be able to use a rectal suppository such as Tigan. It will be important to check your blood glucose every 2 hours and to check for ketones (see page 66). This is a serious situation. You must replace fluids to prevent becoming dehydrated. If diarrhea is severe, taking medication such as Imodium can be helpful if you are able to ingest it without vomiting it up. If you have vomiting and diarrhea for 6 hours and you are unable to keep any fluids down, you should seek medical assistance right away.

WHY DO YOU NEED TO CHECK FOR KETONES?

When you are ill, you must check your urine for ketones (page 66). Ketones are an acid that is a by-product when the body burns fat for fuel instead of carbohydrate. If you take insulin, it means that you need more. No matter which diabetes medication you take, if your body is producing ketones and you don't do anything about it, you can develop a very serious condition called diabetic ketoacidosis (DKA). It can lead to a life-threatening situation and usually requires a trip to the hospital.

Early signs of DKA include high blood glucose levels (higher than 240 mg/dl), moderate to large amounts of ketones in the urine or the blood, headache, muscle and joint aches, and stomach upset. You may only have high blood glucose and ketones, with no other symptoms. It is very important to treat the high blood glucose levels and ketones with insulin and lots of fluids. Usually with extra insulin, the blood glucose and ketone levels will come down. Check the ketone level hourly. If you are unable to lower the blood glucose and clear the ketones with insulin and fluids within 4 hours, seek medical attention. If you slip further into DKA, you may experience shortness of breath, chest pain, and vomiting. If you have these symptoms, you must seek medical care immediately.

WHAT CAN YOU DO ABOUT TRAVELER'S DIARRHEA?

One of your concerns when traveling outside of the United States is getting traveler's diarrhea—a great risk to your health. It usually comes from contact with bacteria-contaminated food or water. The best treatment is prevention. Always drink bottled water. Even brush your teeth with bottled water. Never use ice in drinks. Be sure food is completely cooked. If raw fruits and vegetables cannot be peeled, do not eat them. Do not eat raw vegetables.

If you will be traveling outside of the country, you may want to take Pepto-Bismol daily or antibiotics to prevent traveler's diarrhea from occurring. The correct choice for you will depend on your health needs and where you will be traveling. Talk with your health care provider about this. These same medications are also the ones you would use to treat traveler's diarrhea if you got it (see Table 7-2. *Medications to Prevent and Treat Traveler's Diarrhea*).

Traveler's diarrhea can be categorized into three types. The first type—watery diarrhea—is characterized by explosive, nonbloody stools with nausea, vomiting, abdominal cramping, and fever. This type of diarrhea can affect as many as 60% of travelers. The second type is dysentery. Dysentery affects 15% of travelers. It is characterized by bloody, mucus-laden diarrhea, bowel inflammation, fever, and abdominal pain. Dysentery requires antibiotics and medical care.

Table 7-2. Medications to Prevent and Treat Traveler's Diarrhea

Dose	Dosage	
	For Prevention	For Treatment
*Bismuth subsalicylate (Pepto-Bismol)	2 tablets or 30 ml 4 times per day	2 tablets or 30 ml every hour (don't exceed 8 doses/24 hrs)
**Ciprofloxacin (Cipro)	500 mg per day	500 mg twice daily for 3 days
**Ofloxacin	400 mg per day	400 mg twice daily for 3 days
**Loperamide	Not indicated	4 mg to start, then 2 mg after each unformed stool (not to exceed 16 mg/24 hrs)

There are also other medications to treat traveler's diarrhea. Discuss with your health care provider which ones are best for you to use.

* Over-the-counter medication; no prescription needed. ** Prescription medication.

The third type of traveler's diarrhea is chronic diarrhea. This accounts for fewer than 2% of all cases. Chronic diarrhea often lasts for several weeks. Symptoms include abdominal pain, bloating, fatigue, weight loss, and fever. You need medical evaluation and treatment for chronic diarrhea.

WHAT CAN YOU DO TO AVOID CONSTIPATION?

Drink lots of water—not caffeine drinks such as tea or coffee because they are diuretics and remove water from your body. And not carbonated drinks because they deplete your body of water, too. Eat vegetables. Eat well-washed fruit with the skins on. Eat whole-grains, such as brown rice. Eat some more vegetables. Avoid highly refined foods with lots of white flour, sugar, and salt. Get some exercise. Take your bran flakes with you.

ARE THERE AILMENTS CAUSED BY AN INSULIN PUMP?

If you wear an insulin pump, there is a risk of irritation or infection at the insertion site of your infusion line. You can prevent most site infections by

- washing your hands;
- using a sterile technique you've learned;
- changing your infusion site every other day.

If the site appears irritated when you remove the infusion line, apply warm (not hot) compresses to the area. This increases circulation, which speeds healing. Be sure to insert your new infusion line in an area away from the irritated site. Check it regularly. It may take several days, but gradually, any redness or irritation should go away.

An infusion site may also become infected. An infected site is usually red, warm to the touch, or painful, and it may have drainage. Often the infected area will be hard to the touch. In addition to the care you would provide to an irritated site (keep it clean and apply warm compresses), you need an antibiotic.

You should pack an antibiotic that will treat site infections (see page 35). An infection will often cause high blood glucose levels. Check your blood glucose more frequently to see whether you will need to adjust your insulin. You may also need to check for ketones.

WHAT DO YOU PACK FOR COUGHS AND COLDS?

Be sure to pack medications for treating colds and coughs. Most over-the-counter cold medications are safe for people with diabetes to use, though some can affect your blood glucose level. Many remedies labeled "decongestant" contain ingredients (such as pseudoephedrine) that can raise blood glucose levels and blood pressure. It is best to review this with your health care provider before you travel to be sure these medications will not interfere with other medications that you are taking. Sugar-free cough syrups are available over the counter and by prescription, but they may be difficult to find on the road. Put a bottle of cough syrup in your first aid kit.

WHAT CAN YOU DO ABOUT JET LAG?

Jet lag can occur when you are crossing multiple time zones, so you'll only be affected when you are flying east or west, not north or south. This quick change in time zones prevents your body from adjusting correctly to the new time schedule. The symptoms of jet lag include headaches, constipation, insomnia, nervousness, irritability, sluggishness, and forgetfulness.

There are a few things that you can do to minimize the effects of jet lag. Try to arrive at your destination at bedtime. Get yourself on the schedule of your destination as quickly as possible. Get plenty of rest the day before your departure and when you arrive. Sleep during your flight. Avoid alcohol and caffeine. Drink fluids to avoid becoming dehydrated, because this can make the symptoms of jet lag worse. Drink at least one 8-oz nonalcoholic, decaffeinated beverage every hour of your flight.

WHAT IS A UTI AND WHAT CAN YOU DO ABOUT IT?

People with diabetes are more prone to urinary tract infections (UTIs). Keeping your blood glucose levels well controlled can help prevent UTIs because this allows the body's immune system to ward off bacteria that may enter the urinary tract system. However, UTIs may be caused by another condition. Over time, the muscles of the bladder may become affected by nerve changes caused by diabetes in a condition called neurogenic bladder.

The nerve damage to the bladder does not allow the bladder to empty completely when you urinate. The urine left in the bladder may become contaminated by bacteria. If you have more than two UTIs a year, you will need to see a urologist, a doctor specializing in diseases of the urinary tract. Neurogenic bladder can be treated with medications, so the bladder can empty properly and infections can be prevented. The symptoms of a UTI are:

- Cloudy or bloody urine
- Pain when you urinate

- Constant feeling of pressure and needing to urinate

These symptoms need to be treated with antibiotics. If possible, get a urine culture at a health care clinic before you start taking an antibiotic. The urinalysis will help the health care provider determine the best antibiotic for the bacteria in your urine.

If you are unable to get a culture, start taking the antibiotic with you in your first aid kit. It should be a broad-spectrum antibiotic that kills the usual bacteria that grow in the bladder. For the first 24–48 hours of treatment of a UTI, you often feel pain when you try to urinate. The pain is caused by a contraction or spasm of the urethra, the tube through which urine comes out of the body. If you have this pain, you will want to take, in addition to the antibiotic, a prescription medication called Pyridum. Keep a supply of these tablets in your first aid kit (page 35). Pyridum will stop the spasms of the urethra and work as a local anesthetic on the pain. Be aware that Pyridum will turn your urine a dark red-orange color. In women, it may stain underwear, but a small sanitary pad can help if that is a problem. If you do not have any Pyridum, try urinating in a bathtub filled with clear warm water. This may also decrease the discomfort until the antibiotics have started to work.

Be sure to take all of the antibiotic even if you start feeling better. Be sure to urinate whenever you have the urge. After you complete the antibiotics, get a urine culture done to be sure the bacteria is gone.

Some people find that drinking cranberry juice is helpful in preventing and treating bladder infections. If you drink a glass of cranberry juice, remember to count the amount of carbohydrate in the juice when you are figuring out how much of your diabetes medication to take.

WHAT CAN YOU DO ABOUT VAGINAL INFECTIONS?

Women with diabetes are more likely to get vaginal infections. Vaginal infections can cause pain, itching, and a discharge from the vaginal area. Controlling your blood glucose will help minimize these infections. There are several over-the-counter medications to treat vaginal infections—such as Monistat cream or suppositories—that you can take with you on your trip. If the symptoms do not cease or they come back, be sure to seek medical assistance.

CAN YOU ARRANGE FOR HEALTH CARE BEFORE YOU GO?

Check with your health insurance company to see what coverage you have when you travel out of the area. You will need to know for travel both within the United States as well as out of the country. Be sure you find out the restrictions and requirements and everything that is covered, including paying for flying you home. Medicare does not cover you for overseas travel. If your health insurance does not cover you on your trip, there are many emergency services to help you with health care while traveling (see the box *Emergency Assistance*). Some require you to become a member before you can obtain their services, but most just charge a fee if you need care. Be sure to contact the agencies before beginning your trip, so you are familiar with the services each of them offers.

You May Already Be Covered

Before purchasing travel insurance, check the fine print on your credit card agreement. Your card may already cover illness and special or medical care while you are traveling when you charge the trip to that card. Call your credit card company to see what travel benefits you may have.

You can buy special trip insurance that also covers health care during the trip and a change in flight or cruise schedule to return home. Most have toll-free hotlines, assist you with finding a physician, pay for medical care, and arrange for getting you home. Many of these companies are mentioned in the box *Emergency Assistance*. You must tell the company that you have diabetes and get in writing what they will cover for you and what they will not. For example, Assist-Card can provide translation services and send a doctor to your hotel room if you are sick, cover medical or dental care, and offers accidental death insurance among other services. Be sure to call the benefits department at work and ask if any of these plans are part of your short-term or long-term disability policy. Depending on where you work, your employer may have purchased one of these programs as part of your benefit package. If this is the case, you'll need to get the necessary service code and phone numbers to use the service.

Emergency Assistance

Overseas Citizens' Emergency Center

2201 C Street NW
Washington, DC 20520
1-202-647-5225
www.travel.state.gov

International Association for Medical Assistance to Travelers

1623 Military Road #279
Niagara Falls, NY 14304-1745
1-716-754-4883
www.iamat.org

Free service. Members receive a directory of English-speaking physicians in 125 countries who will provide 24-hour care at reasonable fees.

Assist-Card

1-800-874-2223
www.assist-card.com

International assistance ranging from medical and dental to concierge services. Provides assistance within the U.S. for foreign visitors.

HOTELDOCS

1-800-468-3537
www.hoteldocs.com

Sends an American Medical Association–recruited doctor to your U.S. hotel room within 40 minutes of your call, at any time of day.

International SOS Assistance, Inc.

3600 Horizon Boulevard
Suite 300
Trevose, PA 19053
1-215-942-8000
www.internationalSOS.com

Provides emergency assistance to members. If medical assistance cannot be rendered locally, the traveler will be evacuated to a place with medical facilities.

Travel Guard International

1145 Clark Street
Stevens Point, WI 54481
1-800-826-4919 (U.S.)
1-715-345-0505 (International)
www.travelguard.com

Talk to your travel agent about this service. Offers a 24-hour emergency claims service, emergency assistance, medical expenses, baggage and travel documents coverage, and trip-cancellation insurance. Underwritten by the Insurance Company of North America.

Travelex Insurance Services

PO Box 641070
Omaha, NE 68164-7070
1-888-457-4602
www.travelex.com

Chapter Eight

PLANNING FOR SPECIAL SITUATIONS

Y ou can travel wherever you want to go; there's no reason diabetes should keep you from doing anything you want to do. The key is to plan ahead, so you can be prepared. Try to anticipate problems that may occur and always do the following:

- Know who to call in an emergency.

- Pack enough supplies to be able to manage your diabetes.

- Pack enough food for 24 hours or more, depending on where you're going.

OVERSEAS TRAVEL

Foreign travel can be a challenge if you have not planned ahead. There are United States Consulates in more than 140 countries around the world. They are there to help you, so use them as a resource. Before you travel, contact them either by telephone or through their website (see the box *Consular Information Sheets*) for information regarding your destination. The information sheets include country description, entry requirements, customs regulations, crime information, medical facilities, medical insurance, immunization requirements, and how to register at the U.S. Consulate when you arrive.

Consular Information Sheets

Consular Information Sheets are an excellent resource for anyone traveling abroad. These sheets provide up-to-date information on a wide variety of topics specific to the country you are visiting. You can obtain a copy of Consular Information Sheets by calling 202-647-5225 and speaking with a representative, or by visiting the State Department's travel website at *www.travel.state.gov*.

Foreign languages

If you do not speak the language of the country you are visiting, try to learn a few key phrases before you go. You may need to know how to say: "I have diabetes," "I need sugar," or, "I need a doctor." The Appendix at the back of the book has helpful sentences in Spanish, German, French, Italian, Russian, Japanese, Chinese, and Greek. If you photocopy the sentences or write them down and take them with you, you can read them or point to them if you don't

On the Web

www.tripprep.com

This site contains lots of information on destinations around the world. Topics include information pertaining to hotels, transportation, currency, diplomatic offices, and safety.

www.timeanddates.com

This site provides a world clock and international telephone dialing codes. To get a dialing code, simply type in the city you are calling from, the city you wish to call, and the phone number you wish to call. The website will provide the dialing codes you need.

www.xe.com

This website will help you convert your currency. Type in the amount of currency you wish to convert. Highlight the currency you have and then highlight the currency to which you wish to convert.

feel you can say them. You may also want to take a dictionary or language book with you for help translating other phrases. Ask the concierge or desk clerk at your hotel to write out the address and phone number of the hotel. You can show the address to a taxi driver, or if you are lost, it will assist you in getting back to your hotel.

Always take these along

There are several things to always carry with you:

- Your insulin or diabetes pills
- Blood glucose monitor and supplies
- Foods to treat low blood glucose
- At least one snack (preferably more)

If you need to treat low blood glucose, you do not want to be wandering around looking for a place that has something safe for you to eat. In your cooler or tote, also keep the letter that explains why you are carrying these supplies (see chapter 1).

Global Refund

If you are traveling to any countries that are part of the European Union (EU) and spend at least 125.01 euros in one store in one day, you may be eligible for a tax refund up to 15.5% of your purchase. Go to *www.globalrefund.com* to find out which countries participate and to get more information on how to apply for a refund.

Basically, follow these three steps:

1. If you shop where you see the global tax refund sign in a store and spend at least 125.01 euros in the store in one day, ask for a global refund check.

2. When leaving the country, show the receipts, your purchase, and your passport to the customs officers. They will stamp your global tax refund check.

3. You may collect your refund in cash at the nearby refund office (near customs) or send the check to Global Refund for a bank check sent to your home address or as direct credit to your credit card.

CAMPING

Camping can be a fun way to vacation. Whether you are camping in warm or cold weather, you will need to take special precautions with your insulin. Placing insulin in a cooler will work, but be sure it does not touch the ice. The insulin can freeze and lose potency. If you are camping outdoors in cold weather, don't leave your insulin outside. You can place it in a cooler or a wide-mouth insulated ther-

Diabetes in Thin Air

If you are hiking at higher altitudes, be aware that the symptoms of high altitude sickness (which for people accustomed to living at sea level can occur as low as 9,000 feet) are sometimes similar to the symptoms of low blood glucose. Also be prepared for colder temperatures; if you are cold, your blood glucose may fall. Pay attention to your symptoms and don't guess; go ahead and check your blood glucose level. Also be aware that being at a higher altitude can affect the way your blood glucose meter works. If you know you're going to high altitudes, call your meter company before you go and ask how to adjust your meter to get the correct results under the new conditions.

mos. The thermos will keep it at a steady temperature. Or you can tuck the insulin into your sleeping bag with you, so it won't freeze.

Follows these tips for camping to ensure a safe and fun trip:

☞ Keep all of your diabetes supplies and a complete first aid kit (page 35) in waterproof containers. This will keep your supplies dry, clean, and out of the way of animals and insects. Bring plenty of clothes suitable for the climate—both highs and lows. Also keep ing mind that wherever you go, even in the desert, nights can often get very cool.

☞ Bring extra shoes and socks to change into if yours get wet. If you will be swimming, wear water shoes to protect your feet from injury and infection. In fact, never go barefoot, even in your tent.

☞ Pack a cellular phone for emergencies. Know the phone number and where the nearest emergency center is located.

☞ Use insect repellent to protect yourself from insect bites. Try it out at home to be sure you will not have an allergic reaction or skin irritation to the repellent.

☞ Use sunscreen, a sun hat, sunglasses, and lightweight long-sleeved clothing to protect you from the sun. After-sun creams with aloe or vitamin E are helpful if you've had too much sun.

☞ If you will be hiking, biking, swimming, or getting more exercise than usual, you should check your blood glucose more often because exercise lowers your blood glucose for hours afterward, even into the next day. So after quite a bit of exercise, measure your blood glucose before each meal and at bedtime.

☞ Always carry something with you to treat low blood glucose (see the box on page 51). You may need to take less insulin or adjust the dosage of your diabetes pill or eat some carbohydrate-containing food to balance the beneficial effect exercise has on your blood glucose.

☞ Be sure your companions know your low blood glucose symptoms and what to do if you experience a low, including how to use the glucagon kit (see page 53).

Long trips to the wilderness

Long trips to remote areas require serious planning, but they can be—and have been—done by people with diabetes! In addition to the health visits, immunizations, and supplies, you must know the area in which you will be traveling. Talk with others who have done the same or similar trips. Talk with the company or travel agency that will be setting up the trip. Learn from others what to expect when you get there. Some of the questions you need to ask are:

• What facilities will be available?

• How will you obtain food?

• What types of food are available?

• Will there be storage available for your insulin?

• What medical facilities are available?

• How far will you be from a medical facility?

• What assistance can you expect if a medical emergency occurs?

Many of these trips are so remote that you may not see anyone but your traveling companions for long periods. All of these questions need to be answered before you take your trip. And at least one of your companions needs to know how to recognize and treat low blood glucose, including how to use a glucagon kit.

After your questions are answered, it is time to plan what you will need to take. All the advice for general traveling tips apply. The difference is that you have no way to obtain more diabetes supplies if something happens to yours. Take great care in packing and handling your diabetes supplies (in several bags) and keep them with you. It will be important to pack snacks that you can divide into single servings and seal so that they do not attract animals or insects.

SCUBA DIVING

Scuba diving is a favorite pastime of many people who visit warm tropical areas.

Scuba Diving Guidelines

1. The dive should follow a meal. Always measure your blood glucose several times before you dive. It should be at least 150 mg/dl and not dropping.

2. If your blood glucose before the dive is lower than 150 mg/dl, you need to eat or drink 5 g of glucose (5 g of carbohydrate) for every 25 mg/dl it is below 150 mg/dl. Try carbohydrates such as milk, fruit juice, or glucose tablets/liquid.

3. You and your diving partner must carry liquid glucose or gel during the dive and use it as needed.

4. Measure your blood glucose right after the dive and eat or drink more carbohydrates if you need them.

5. Always dive with a companion who understands how to recognize and treat low blood glucose. Before you're under water, decide on a way to communicate that you may be developing low blood glucose.

6. You should have good blood glucose control during the days you plan to go diving.

7. Don't drink alcohol in the 24 hours before diving or during diving activities.

There is no reason that you cannot learn to scuba dive. First, you need to take a course and become certified in scuba diving. Then, there are several precautions that you need to follow to make diving safe (see the box *Scuba Diving Guidelines*).

Your blood glucose should be above 150 mg/dl. If blood glucose is less than 150 mg/dl or dropping, take 5 g of glucose (see the box *Over-the-Counter Products to Treat Low Blood Glucose* on page 51) for every 25 mg/dl it is below 150 mg/dl. You and your dive partner should both carry liquid or gel glucose in a tube during every dive. Agree on a low blood glucose signal. Be very aware that swimming in cold water will cause your blood glucose to drop quickly, so be alert to symptoms of low blood glucose. Don't drink alcohol for 24 hours before the time of the dive.

Be sure to take your diving certification card when you travel. When you complete an application, you will be asked about your diabetes. Bring along a letter from your doctor indicating their recommendations for you to be able to dive safely (see the *Example of a Scuba Diving Letter*).

Example of a Scuba Diving Letter

Date:

To Whom It May Concern:

RE: (*Your name*)

Mr. (*Your Name*) has diabetes and takes insulin. He has successfully completed a certified diving course. We have many patients who successfully scuba dive and we recommend that:

1. The patient completes a certified diving course.

2. The patient monitors his blood glucose before each dive. Blood glucose should be above 150 mg/dl before a dive. If it is less than 150 mg/dl, he should ingest 5 g of glucose for every 25 mg/dl under 150 mg/dl.

3. The patient carries liquid or gel glucose during dives.

4. The patient follows the recommended dive tables.

5. The patient should dive with a companion who is able to treat low blood glucose (hypoglycemia).

6. The patient should not drink any alcohol for 24 hours before the time of the dive.

If you have any questions, please contact me.

Sincerely yours,

(*Provider's signature*)

Health care provider's name:

_____

Address:

_____

Telephone numbers:

_____

APPENDIX. FOREIGN PHRASE BOOK

SPANISH

Please help me. I have diabetes.
Por favór ayudenme. Tengo diabetes.

May I please have some sugar or
fruit juice or Coke?
**¿Me podría asistir con azúcar, o
jugo de frutas, o una coca-cola?**

My blood sugar is too low.
Mi nivél de azúcar está muy bajo.

I must have something to eat.
Necesito comer algo con urgencia.

Where is the American Consulate?
**¿Donde está el Consulado
Americano?**

Where is the hospital?
¿Donde está el hospital?

Where may I buy medicine?
¿Donde podría comprar medicina?

Where is the grocery store?
¿Donde está el mercado?

Where is a telephone?
¿Donde está el teléfono?

Where is the hotel?
¿Donde está el hotel?

Where may I buy batteries?
¿Donde podría comprar baterias?

I need some milk to drink.
Necesito tomar leche.

I need to buy some insulin.
Necesito comprar insulina.

I need to buy some insulin syringes.
Necesito comprar jeringas.

GERMAN

Please help me. I have diabetes.
Helfen Sie mir bitte, ich bin ein Diabetiker.

May I please have some sugar or fruit juice or Coke?
Koennten Sie mir bitte etwas Zucker, einen Fruchtesaft oder eine Cola geben?

My blood sugar is too low.
Mein Blutzucker ist zu niedrig.

I must have something to eat.
Ich muss etwas zu essen haben.

Where is the American Consulate?
Wo ist das Amerikanische Konsulat?

Where is the hospital?
Wo ist das Hospital?

Where may I buy medicine?
Wo kann ich Medikamente einkaufen?

Where is the grocery store?
Wo ist ein Lebensmittelgeschaeft?

Where is the telephone?
Wo ist ein Telefon?

Where is the hotel?
Wo ist das Hotel?

Where may I buy batteries?
Wo gibt es Batterien zu kaufen?

I need some milk to drink.
Koennten Sie mir bitte etwas milch geben?

I need to buy some insulin.
Ich muss das Insulin kaufen.

Can I buy diabetic supplies?
Kann ich diabetiker bedorf kaufen?

FRENCH

Please help me. I have diabetes.
Aidez-moi. Je suis diabetique.

May I please have some sugar or fruit juice or Coke?
Pouvez vous me donner du sucre, un jus de fruit ou un Coca Cola ?

My blood sugar is too low.
Mon taux de sucre dans le sang est trop bas. Je suis en etat d'hypoglycemie.

I must have something to eat.
Je dois manger quelque chose.

I need some milk to drink.
J'ai besoin de boire du lait.

I need to buy some insulin.
J'ai besoin d'acheter de l'insuline.

I need to buy some insulin syringes.
J'ai besoin d'acheter des seringues pour l'insuline.

Where is the American Consulate?
Ou se trouve le consulat des Etats-Unis?

Where is the hospital?
Ou se trouve l'hopital?

Where may I buy medicine? Where is a phramacy?
Ou puis-je acheter des medicaments?
Ou est la pharmacie?

Where is the grocery store?
Ou est le supermarché?

Where is the telephone?
Ou est le téléphone?

Where is the hotel?
Ou est l' hotel?

Where may I buy batteries?
Ou puis-je acheter des piles?

ITALIAN

Please help me. I have diabetes.
Aiutatemi-ho il diabete. Soffro il diabete.

May I please have some sugar or fruit juice or Coke?
Per favore potrei avere un po' di zucchero, un succo di frutta o una coca cola?

My blood sugar is too low.
Ho la glicemia troppo bassa.

I must have something to eat.
Devo mangiare qualcosa.

I need some milk to drink.
Devo bere del latte.

I need to buy some insulin.
Devo comprare la insulina per il diabete.

I need to buy some insulin syringes.
Mi occorrono le siringhe da insulina.

Where is the American Consulate?
Dov'è il consolato americano?

Where is the hospital?
Dov'è l'ospedale?

Where may I buy medicine? Where is a pharmacy?
Dov'è posso comprare della medicina?
Dov'è una farmacia?

Where is the grocery store?
Dov'è un supermercato o un negozio alimentare?

Where is the telephone?
Dov'è c'è un telefono?

Where is the hotel?
Dov'è l'albergo?

Where may I buy batteries?
Dov'è posso comprare le pile?

RUSSIAN

Please help me. I have diabetes.

Pomogeetye minye, pozhalooista.
Ya diabetik.
Помогите мне, пожалуйста.
Я диабетик.

May I please have some sugar or fruit
juice or Coke?

Mozhno sakhar, sok eelee koka-koloo?
Можно сахар, сок или кока-колу?

My blood sugar is too low.

Oo menya nizki ooroven sakhara v krovee.
У меня низкий уровень сахара в
крови.

I must have something to eat.

Minye nada poyest.
Мне надо поесть.

Where is the American Consulate?

Gidye amerikanskoye konsoolstvo?
Где американское консульство?

Where is the hospital?
Gidye bolnitsa?
Где больница?

Where may I buy medicine?
Gidye koopeet lekarstvo?
Где купить лекарство?

Where is the grocery store?
Gidye nakhoditsya prodooktovee magazeen?
Где находится продуктовый магазин?

Where is a telephone?
Gidye ya magoo naitee telefon?
Где я могу найти телефон?

Where is the _____ Hotel?
Gidye gostinitsa _____?
Где гостиница _____?

Where may I buy batteries?
Gidye mozhno koopeet akoomoolyatoree?
Где можно купить аккумуляторы?

I need some milk to drink.

Minye nada veepeet moloka.

Мне надо выпить молока.

I need to buy some insulin.

Minye nada koopeet insulin.

Мне надо купить инсулин.

I need to buy some insulin syringes.

Minye nada koopeet shpreetz dilya insulina.

Мне надо купить шприц для инсулина.

JAPANESE

Please help me. I have diabetes.

Watashi wa toonyoobyoo desu.

Tedasuke shite tadake nasu ka.

私 は 糖 尿 病 で す.手 助 け し て い た だ け ま す か.

May I please have some sugar or fruit juice or Coke?

Satoo to jyuusu to koora wa doko desu ka?

砂 糖 と ジ ュ ー ス と コ ー ラ は 何 処 で す か.

May I please have some milk?

Miruku o ne ga i shimasu?

ミ ル ク お 願 い し ま す.

My blood sugar is too low.

Watashi no ketochi wa totem tekui desu.

私 の 血 糖 値 は と て も て く い で す.

I must have something to eat.

Ima nani ga taberu shitsuku go orimasu.

い ま な に が 食 べ る し つ く が あ り ま す.

Where is the American Consulate?

Amerika no ryoojikan wa doko desu ka?

アメリカ の 大使館 は 何処 で
す か .

Where is the hospital?

Byooin wa doko desu ka?

病院 は 何処 で す か .

Where may I buy medicine?

Doko de kusuri ga kae masu ka?

何処 で く す り が 買 え ま す か .

Where is the grocery store?

Suapoa maaketto wa doko desu ka?

ス ー パ は 何処 で す か .

Where is the telephone?

Denwa wa doko desu ka?

電話 は 何処 で す か .

Where is the _____ Hotel?

_____ hoteru wa doko desu ka?

.... ホ テ ル は 何処 で す か .

Where may I buy batteries?

Doko de denchi ga kaemasuka?

何 処 で 電 池 が 買 え ま す か .

I need to buy some insulin.

Doko de insulin ga kaemasuka.

何 処 で イ ン ス リ ン が 買 え ま
す か .

I need to buy some insulin syringes.

Doko de insulin chushia ga kaemasuka.

何 処 で イ ン ス リ ン 注 射 針 が 買
え ま す か .

CHINESE

Please help me. I have diabetes.

Qíng bāngzhù wǒ. Wǒ yǒu tángnìaobìng.

請 幫 助 我. 我 有 糖 尿 病.

May I please have some sugar or
fruit juice or Coca Cola?

**Qíng gěi wǒ yī xiē táng, hùo gǔozhī, hùo
shì kěkǒukělè hǎo ma?**

請 給 我 一 些 糖, 或 果 汁,
或 是 可 口 可 樂 好 嗎?

May I please have some milk?

Qíng gěi wǒ yī xiē níunǎi hǎo ma?

請 給 我 一 些 牛 奶 好 嗎?

My blood sugar is too low.

Wǒ de xǔetáng hěn dī.

我 的 血 糖 很 低.

I must have something to eat.

Wǒ bìxū chī dǐan dōngxī.

我 必 須 吃 點 東 西.

Where is the American Consulate?

Qǐngwèn měiguó lǐngshìguǎn zài nálǐ?

請 問 美 國 領 事 館 在 那 裏?

Where is the hospital?

Qǐngwèn yīyùan zài nálǐ?

請 問 醫 院 在 那 裏?

Where may I buy medicine?

Qǐngwèn zài nálǐ kěyǐ mǎi yào?

請 問 在 那 裏 可 以 買 藥 ?

Where is the grocery store?

Qǐngwèn chāoshì zài nálǐ?

請 問 超 市 在 那 裏?

Where is a telephone?

Qǐngwèn dìanhùa zài nálǐ?

請 問 電 話 在 那 裏?

Where is the _____ Hotel?

Qǐngwèn _____ lǚguǎn zài nálǐ?

請 問....... 旅 館 在 那 裏?

Where may I buy batteries?

Qǐngwèn zài nálǐ kěyǐ mǎi diànchí?

請 問 在 那 裏 可 以 買 電 池?

I need to buy some insulin.

Wǒ xūyào mǎi xiē yídǎosù zhìjì.

我 需 要 買 些 胰 島 素 製 劑.

I need to buy some insulin syringes.

Wǒ xūyào mǎi xiē yídǎosù zhùshèzhēn.

我 需 要 買 些 胰 島 素 注 射 針.

GREEK

I have diabetes.

Eho zaharo.

Εψω ζαχαρο.

I need sugar, orange juice, or a coca cola.

The'lo zahaou, portokalada,

l ena coca cola.

Θελω ζαχαρη, πορτοκαλαδα η ενα γλνκο πιοτο.

INDEX

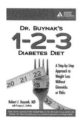
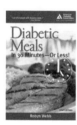
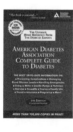

About the American Diabetes Association

The American Diabetes Association is the nation's leading voluntary health organization supporting diabetes research, information, and advocacy. Its mission is to prevent and cure diabetes and to improve the lives of all people affected by diabetes. The American Diabetes Association is the leading publisher of comprehensive diabetes information. Its huge library of practical and authoritative books for people with diabetes covers every aspect of self-care—cooking and nutrition, fitness, weight control, medications, complications, emotional issues, and general self-care.

To order American Diabetes Association books: Call 1-800-232-6733. Or log on to *http://store.diabetes.org*

To join the American Diabetes Association: Call 1-800-806-7801. *www.diabetes.org/membership*

For more information about diabetes or ADA programs and services: Call 1-800-342-2383. E-mail: AskADA@diabetes.org or log on to *www.diabetes.org*

To locate an ADA/NCQA Recognized Provider of quality diabetes care in your area: *www.ncqa.org/dprp*

To find an ADA Recognized Education Program in your area: Call 1-888-232-0822. *www.diabetes.org/recognition/education.asp*

To join the fight to increase funding for diabetes research, end discrimination, and improve insurance coverage: Call 1-800-342-2383. *www.diabetes.org/advocacy*

To find out how you can get involved with the programs in your community: Call 1-800-342-2383. See below for program Web addresses.

- *American Diabetes Month:* educational activities aimed at those diagnosed with diabetes—month of November. *www.diabetes.org/ADM*
- *American Diabetes Alert:* annual public awareness campaign to find the undiagnosed—held the fourth Tuesday in March. *www.diabetes.org/alert*
- *The Diabetes Assistance & Resources Program (DAR):* diabetes awareness program targeted to the Latino community. *www.diabetes.org/DAR*
- *African American Program:* diabetes awareness program targeted to the African American community. *www.diabetes.org/africanamerican*
- *Awakening the Spirit: Pathways to Diabetes Prevention & Control:* diabetes awareness program targeted to the Native American community. *www.diabetes.org/awakening*

To find out about an important research project regarding type 2 diabetes: *www.diabetes.org/ada/research.asp*

To obtain information on making a planned gift or charitable bequest: Call 1-888-700-7029. *www.diabetes.org/ada/plan.asp*

To make a donation or memorial contribution: Call 1-800-342-2383. *www.diabetes.org/ada/cont.asp*